The Discipline of Nursing

AN INTRODUCTION

Fourth Edition

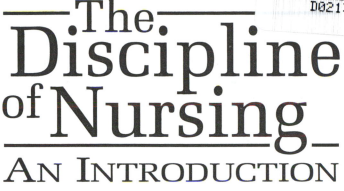

Margaret O'Bryan Doheny, RN, PhD, ONC
Associate Professor, School of Nursing
Kent State University, Kent, Ohio

Christina Benson Cook, RN, PhD
Assistant Professor, School of Nursing
Kent State University, Kent, Ohio

Mary Constance Stopper, RN, MEd, MSN
Associate Professor and Assistant Dean, School of Nursing
Kent State University, Kent, Ohio
Doctoral Candidate, College of Education
The University of Akron, Akron, Ohio

Appleton & Lange
Stamford, Connecticut

Copyright © 1997 by Appleton & Lange
A Simon & Schuster Company
Copyright © 1992, 1987 by Appleton & Lange
Copyright © 1982 by Brady Communications, Inc.

97 98 99 00 01 / 10 9 8 7 6 5 4 3 2 1

Prentice Hall International (UK) Limited, *London*
Prentice Hall of Australia Pty. Limited, *Sydney*
Prentice Hall Canada, Inc., *Toronto*
Prentice Hall Hispanoamericana, S.A., *Mexico*
Prentice Hall of India Private Limited, *New Delhi*
Prentice Hall of Japan, Inc., *Tokyo*
Simon & Schuster Asia Pte. Ltd., *Singapore*
Editora Prentice Hall do Brasil Ltda., *Rio de Janeiro*
Prentice Hall, *Upper Saddle River, New Jersey*

Library of Congress Cataloging-in-Publication Data
Doheny, Margaret O'Bryan
    The discipline of nursing : an introduction / Margaret O'Bryan
Doheny, Christina Benson Cook, Mary Constance Stopper. -- 4th ed.
        p. cm.
    Includes index.
    ISBN 0-8385-1716-1 (pbk. : alk. paper)
    1. Nursing--Vocational guidance. 2. Nursing. I. Cook, Christina
Benson. II. Stopper, Mary Constance. III. Title.
    [DNLM: 1. Nursing. WY 16 D655d 1997]
RT82.D63   1997
610.73'06'9--dc20
DNLM/DLC
for Library of Congress   96-20875

Acquisitions Editor: David P. Carroll
Production Editor: Lisa M. Guidone
Cover Designer: Michael J. Kelly
Interior Designer: Janice Barsevich Bielawa

ISBN 0-8385-1716-1

90000

PRINTED IN THE UNITED STATES OF AMERICA

Contents

Preface

It is now common to find schools of nursing offering a beginning-level course to introduce students to the discipline of professional nursing. These courses focus on the theoretical aspect of nursing rather than the practice aspect. Often they are survey courses based on the individual school's curriculum or instructor's viewpoint. Students frequently enter these courses with questions about the practice aspect of nursing. These questions usually include "What does a nurse do?" and "When do we learn how to care for a patient?", whereas questions reflecting nursing as a discipline are infrequently raised. The primary focus of this text is to familiarize students with the various aspects of nursing as a discipline.

Students entering nursing today come from diverse personal as well as educational backgrounds. These students possess a combination of both accurate knowledge and misconceptions about nursing. Such misconceptions are understandable, since the nursing profession itself is facing the challenge of identifying its own body of knowledge, educational preparation, and the changing role within the health care delivery system.

Nursing has a dynamic nature and is in continual interaction with a multifaceted, changing environment. Perceptions of health and perspectives of persons in relation to health continue to evolve. Personal and professional development in response to the dynamic nature of nursing, the changing environment, and evolving perceptions of health and of persons has given impetus to the revision of this text. Suggestions from students and colleagues who have used this text have been incorporated in this fourth edition.

The fourth edition is designed to assist the student to conceptualize and clarify nursing as a discipline. Several chapters have been revised to meet this objective. In the first chapter, we describe discipline as the body of knowledge and theory and explain why it is essential for professional nursing. The central concepts to the discipline of person, environment, and health are discussed. Chapter 2 introduces the student to the various theoretical approaches to nursing. The discipline of nursing and the concepts of person, environment, and health are described by various nurse theorists. The historical development of nursing and nursing education is developed in Chapter 3. Themes such as social issues, the role of women, religion and spirituality, influence of the military, and increased technology are discussed in relation to the nursing history. Since educational development in nursing is strongly tied to our historical development, we have included the development of various educational programs in this chapter.

Professional development of nursing is presented in Chapter 4. Material on socialization and role development has been included in this chapter. It is our intent that students develop an understanding of nursing from a professional viewpoint as well as their own understanding of nursing and nursing practice. Chapter 5 has been updated to reflect the current changes in health care delivery including the health care system, influences on the system, health care services, and health care providers. Chapter 6 examines the implementation of the role of the nurse in various settings of the health care delivery system. Aspects of nursing practice, nursing process, and the role of nursing in various settings such as primary, secondary, and tertiary care are presented. Different areas of specialization and opportunities for nursing practice are discussed, as are the enhanced opportunities for nurses at the advanced practice level. The chapter on nursing evaluation and research is developed within the framework that research is essential to validate knowledge, develop new nursing knowledge, and augment nursing practice. We feel strongly that beginning students need to have an appreciation for research and understand the relationship between research and theory development. Evaluation is addressed in terms of structure, process, and outcome. Ethical and legal considerations in Chapter 8 have been updated to reflect the new licensing and credentialing processes.

Specific examples throughout the text have been revised and updated to reflect the focus of nursing on health promotion. The basic format of the text has been maintained, including student objectives, questions to think about, terms to know, a glossary, and questions for discussion.

Peggy Doheny
Chris Cook
Connie Stopper

1 CHAPTER

The Discipline of Nursing

▸ **Objectives**

After studying the chapter, the student will be able to:

1. Describe the components of theory, practice, and research as they relate to the discipline of nursing.
2. List the foundational components or central concepts of the discipline of nursing.
3. State her or his own beliefs about humankind.
4. Describe some of the environmental influences on health.
5. List several definitions of health.
6. State four influences on health.

▸ **Questions to think about before reading the chapter**

- What does it mean to refer to nursing as a discipline?
- How is research relevant to nursing?
- What are your personal beliefs or philosophy about humankind?
- What are some factors that influence health?
- What factors define health?
- Do you consider yourself to be a healthy person? Why?
- Can you recognize different degrees of health in yourself? How?

▸ **Terms to know**

Becoming	Culture
Boundaries	Diagnosis-related group (DRG)
Concept	Discipline
Conceptual models	Environment
Consumer	Health

Holistic	Postmodernism
Kluckhohn, Clyde	Practice
Maslow, Abraham	Research
Metaparadigm	Rogers, Carl
Paradigm	Self-actualization
Patient's Bill of Rights	Social Policy Statement
Person	Society
Philosophical approach	Stress

▶ *Introduction*

This chapter describes nursing as a discipline with a theoretical body of knowledge that provides a foundation for practice. Nursing is continually refined with the support of research. Theory is presented as the outcome of a cognitive process resulting from knowledge development and providing direction to nursing practice. Nursing theorists' ideas are introduced as examples of theory development in nursing. Research is discussed as a means of developing and testing theory. The practice component of nursing is described as a vehicle for implementation of theory as well as validation and impetus for research.

This chapter will provide a basis for discussion of the major theoretical approaches to nursing presented in Chapter 2 and will provide a basis for understanding of the historical development of nursing in Chapter 3.

FRAMEWORK OF NURSING

Nursing has emerged as a unique and integrated discipline that encompasses both science (e.g., biology, physiology, anatomy) and the arts and humanities (e.g., sociology, philosophy, psychology, art, history, and language). Although nursing shares some of the knowledge of the disciplines of medicine, sociology, biology, psychology, and other fields, unique theory and concept development has occurred within nursing. Continued testing of the concepts of other disciplines reformulated to relate to nursing and the testing of nursing theories will advance nursing as a science and a discipline. In addition, the integration, expansion, and use of these areas in providing total patient care distinguish nursing as a discipline. This idea of nursing being a unique and separate discipline was first addressed by Florence Nightingale in 1859. Thus, nursing is an evolving discipline.

Most nursing leaders refer to nursing as both a science and an art. The science of nursing involves a "body of abstract knowledge" that has been arrived at through scientific research and logical analysis. The body of knowledge can be communicated and replicated through research. The art of nursing involves the creative use of this knowledge in service to people.

Greene (1979) also suggests that nursing is both an art and a science. There is some thought in nursing that the science of nursing and the art of nursing can best be addressed through the use of different research methodologies (i.e., qualitative and quantitative research designs). These research designs will be discussed more in Chapter 7.

Art can be described as a creative act or thought process based on theory, personal knowledge, or esthetics. Science is public and involves observable phenomena and theories or abstractions. It does not involve personal knowing or esthetics. Both science and art are dependent on the individual's or society's world view for direction and expression.

Nursing science can be thought of as the theories or the knowledge base of nursing, while nursing art can be viewed as the creative application of that knowledge base to individuals, groups, and cultures. These are complementary ideas, and the use of one does not negate the use of another. This text will view the discipline of nursing as the body of knowledge having a variety of theories. Both art and science incorporate ethical issues into their realm of knowing and acting in reality. The perspective of a discipline provides a broader, more accurate way of viewing nursing than from a view that emphasizes task performance. Nursing practice derives from nursing's knowledge and is the application of nursing's theory. Theory relies on research as well as contributing to it. Theory is continually changed and expanded through research.

DISCIPLINE OF NURSING

The word discipline has often been associated with order, training for self-control, and even punishment. The concept of discipline is much broader than these narrow definitions. Webster's dictionary defines discipline as a branch of knowledge or learning, training that develops self-control, and following a system of rules. Donaldson & Crowley (1978, p. 113) characterize discipline as "a unique perspective, a distinct way of viewing all phenomena, which ultimately defines the limits and nature of its inquiry." A discipline, in general, is a method or way to view an occurrence in a particular manner. Each discipline has a knowledge base that is distinct from that of other disciplines and provides a foundation for practice. The primary purpose of a discipline is the pursuit and development of knowledge. This knowledge base is enhanced and developed through research and provides direction for practice.

Nursing is referred to as a profession and a discipline. It integrates practice and theory and it is expanded and developed through research. Distinctive features are considered when describing nursing as a discipline. Its limits, boundaries, or parameters must be defined. The overall perspective of the practice must also be delineated. By describing the discipline in such a manner, nursing is distinguished from nondisciplines. The concept of professionalism will be discussed in Chapter 4.

Theory

The discipline of nursing has emerged from the needs of a complex, ever-changing society and is a unique interrelationship of art and science. Nursing is a service-oriented profession that finds expression in clinical practice. Essential to any practice is the theory that supports it. Historically, the word theory is derived from the Greek word *theoria*, meaning abstract thought. The Greeks used theory to help explain their world in a logical manner rather than using explanations based on the supernatural.

Theory involves intellectual operations and is constituted of facts, principles, and concepts that are arranged to show their interrelatedness. A theory describes something, a happening or a phenomenon. In more common terms, a theory is used to explain phenomena and organize ideas and knowledge. Theory development enables one to describe, explain, predict, control, or prescribe phenomena of interest. For a theory to be nursing theory, it must be about phenomena that are of nursing's focus of inquiry, not those of another discipline.

Dickoff & Wiedenbach (1968) have identified four levels of theory development: factor-isolating, factor-relating, situation-relating, and situation-producing theories. The factor-isolating theories are the beginning steps for defining a discipline and are often viewed as a pretheoretical phase of theory development. Factor-relating is a more descriptive stage and shows relationships within the theory concepts and propositions. Situation-relating theories are predictive and explanatory. The highest level of theory development is situation-producing, which allows for control and manipulation of variables. This is the level suggested for nursing theory development and includes the assumption of lower-level theories within the discipline.

Theory building is a process that links facts, principles, and concepts together logically. Propositions link concepts into statements. This can be illustrated by the following example. Communication is a **concept** or label representing the sending and receiving of a message from one person to another. There are many facts and principles involved in communication. For instance, at least two people are necessary for communication to occur, and there must be a vehicle for communicating. Nurse and client are two other concepts. The concepts of communication, nurse, and client may be linked together in the following manner. When certain skills are used to facilitate communication between nurse and client in a goal-directed manner, the therapeutic communication process occurs. In the preceding statement, several concepts have been identified and linked together. Concept linking is essential to theory development.

Another example of the interrelationship of facts, principles, and concepts in building theory and applying it to nursing practice is the common procedure of hand washing. A basic principle is that friction applied to the skin decreases the pathogens (disease-producing organisms) on the skin surface. Another related principle is that soap breaks surface tension and emulsifies fats. These two principles can be linked together to form part of an integrated framework related to medical asepsis (the absence of pathogens).

Asepsis is an example of a concept, a label or naming of an object to be studied. Concepts related to asepsis are health and client. When the principles of asepsis are followed, the client's health is promoted. Other common concepts identified in nursing include pain, self-care, stress, and crisis.

Nursing is a practice or applied discipline. Glaser & Strauss (1967) have identified four criteria for practice theory development. A practice theory must closely fit the area in which it is to be used, be general enough to cover diverse practice situations, be understandable to the practitioners using it, and allow control over changing situations.

Theory development is essential to nursing **practice** in that it describes, predicts, controls, and explains phenomena of interest to nurses. Theory validates, enhances, and improves nursing practice. It promotes understanding and explanation of the phenomena and gives rise to the body of knowledge. Theory development follows a logical progression and contributes to nursing's autonomy and identity. Historically, nursing has not placed enough emphasis on the theoretical basis of practice. Theory is intrinsic to practice, and practice continues to validate theory. Theory and practice are integral to one another.

Specifying, defining, and classifying facts, principles, and concepts are the first stages of theory development as described by Jacox (1974) and form the basis for higher stages of theory development, which are relating and interrelating concepts. Concepts are linked to explain approaches to nursing care logically and to predict the outcome of care. In the past, nursing skills were taught because they were "routine" functions of staff nurses. Nurses often functioned with implied or apprenticeship information as a basis for their actions rather than actual facts and principles. If a particular way of doing something seemed to help one nurse, it was passed on to other nurses without study or research of the actual outcomes. Although this transmission of unverified information did in some cases advance nursing practice, it also gave rise to a number of old wives' tales. The discipline of nursing has evolved from unverified information as a basis for practice to development of a solid knowledge or theoretical base that provides rationales for the use of skills (affective, cognitive, and psychomotor) needed for nursing practice.

The concepts central to the discipline are organized in frameworks called **conceptual models.** Conceptual models have been developed to define nursing's central concepts and varied world views. A conceptual model provides a frame of reference for members of the discipline. The framework identifies areas for focus and speculation and determines how the world is viewed. The terms *conceptual frameworks* or *models* and *theoretical frameworks* or *models* differ in several ways. A conceptual framework or model is broad, global, and cannot be subjected to empirical validation. A theoretical framework or model is more specific and narrower in scope and may be amenable to research. Often conceptual models provide the groundwork from which theory is developed. There may be several theories related to a specific conceptual framework. Within nursing, Orem, Rogers, King, Roy, and other theorists have developed conceptual frameworks or models. King and Roy are two theorists who have also developed theoretical frameworks or models from their conceptualizations. These theorists will be discussed in further detail in Chapter 2.

Grand nursing theories provide a broad perspective for looking at nursing phenomena. Jacox (1974) proposes the development of middle-range theories for nursing, since the focus of nursing changes in response to societal needs. As these theories become no longer useful or accurate, they can be modified to fit the new need or knowledge base. Merton, an often quoted sociologist, emphasized the need for middle-range theory development for discipline advancement (1977). Some examples of middle-range theories are those related to pain alleviation, immobility, and stress management. Some authors have developed partial theories. Partial theories deal with a very narrow range of phenomena and are often summarizations of isolated observations (Fawcett, 1984).

In reviewing the development of the concepts and theories prevalent in the discipline of nursing today, many influential factors can be identified. Examples of some factors are the status of nursing at a particular time in history, the experience and education of nurses who developed the theory, and factors and attitudes in society that influence health care and nursing practice. A strong belief held by many nurses today is that the need for continued theory development and testing in contemporary nursing practice is essential.

Practice

In discussing an applied discipline, it is essential that the basis of practice is the knowledge base emphasized. Conceptual and theoretical frameworks provide a way in which to view the person, environment, and health and organize facts, principles, and theories for provision of nursing care. Many societal factors interface with nursing to shape its practice, but it is nursing that must continuously evaluate these factors in view of what is healthiest for the client and the environment. From this ongoing evaluation, nurses continually redefine the practice of nursing. Chapter 6 specifically addresses the area of nursing practice.

Research

Theory and practice have been discussed as components of the discipline of nursing. **Research**, the third component, provides a basis for practice and development of new nursing science. Research is a systematic method of inquiry. The purposes of research include the discovery or validation of knowledge, thus establishing a knowledge base to be used in practice. Research, in contributing to the development of theory for practice, helps to foster the development of the discipline of nursing and to meet the increasingly complex health care needs of our society.

In the past, nurses have observed other nurses in an attempt to look at the components and makeup of the profession. Nurses are now using research as a method for the analysis and resolution of nursing care problems and determination of client care needs. Research is also used to clarify theoretical concepts and build nursing knowledge. Nursing practice is improved and enhanced through the clarification of concepts and increases in nursing's knowledge base.

Nursing research has become vital to the development of the profession and to the practice of nursing. Research leads to the advancement of nursing and nursing theory, changes in nursing practice, and improvement in client care. The component of research will be discussed further in Chapter 7.

DEFINITION OF NURSING

Nursing has frequently been defined in terms of tasks completed or performed, such as caring for the ill, administering medications and treatments, and helping those in need. Definitions of a nurse have often been confused with definitions of nursing; thus, personal characteristics such as knowledge, calmness and coolness in emergencies, a pleasant personality, and the female gender have often been used to define nursing. These characteristics may in fact define or describe certain attributes of a nurse, but they do not define nursing, and they are specific and limiting.

In 1980, the American Nurses Association (ANA) published *Nursing: A Social Policy Statement,* which defined nursing as "the diagnosis and treatment of human responses to actual or potential health problems." Most recently, the ANA has reaffirmed the profession's commitment to the care of individuals, groups, and communities both healthy and ill (1995). The ANA's current statement about the definition of nursing encompasses four essential aspects: "attention to the full range of human experiences and responses to health and illness without restriction to a problem-focused orientation; integration of objective data with knowledge gained from an understanding of the patient or group's subjective experience; application of scientific knowledge to the processes of diagnosis and treatment; and provision of a caring relationship that facilitates health and healing (1995, p.6)."

In all the definitions of nursing, the client is the central focus— the physical, emotional, psychological, social, and spiritual dimensions of the individual. Definitions of nursing involve goals aimed at nursing's role in promoting the health and optimal well-being of individuals, family, or other social systems. The changing definitions reveal that nursing is progressing from the traditional cure concept of caring for ill individuals to a concept that includes prevention of illness and health promotion and maintenance in caring for individuals, their families, and society. It is projected that future systems of care will focus most heavily on the promotion of health and well-being. Nursing enhances the strengths of an individual by viewing the total person, rather than a group of separate entities. For example, when caring for an individual who has a problem of weight control, the nurse must consider diet, lifestyle, support systems, activity levels, and physical status such as height and body build. Nurses look for the area of strength in each client in order to increase self-esteem and focus on the positive and healthy aspects of the individual. A client is no longer viewed as an illness that needs to be treated or as an entity separate from family, environment, and significant others. The family is encouraged to become involved in the client's health and to express their concerns and fears. The nurse looks at all aspects of the client's life in order to promote healthy lifestyles and prevent the occurrence or recurrence of illness. The physical, psychological, social, emotional, and spiritual dimensions of the individual are considered in helping the person reach and maintain an optimal health level.

FOUNDATIONS OF THE DISCIPLINE OF NURSING

As previously discussed, the concepts central to **discipline** are organized in frameworks called conceptual models. Conceptual models have been developed to reaffirm nursing's central concepts and varied world views. A conceptual model provides a frame of reference for members of the discipline. The framework identifies areas for focus and speculation and determines how the world is viewed.

Recently, nursing authors have been discussing nursing's central concepts within the framework of **metaparadigm** and **paradigm.** The term *paradigm* is usually used in connection with the philosophical writings of Thomas Kuhn (1970). Kuhn has identified a paradigm as a model, pattern, or world view that is based on two characteristics of achievement. These two essential characteristics are attraction of a group of people away from the existing or current model of belief and being open-ended enough to allow for problem solving by this group of persons. Paradigms can be in preparadigm and postparadigm, debating over what will be the essential problems to be addressed and what will be the accepted methods for problem solving. No agreement is usually reached in these debates, but they do serve to clarify differing schools of thought. The postparadigm period occurs after the paradigm has been accepted. Scientific progress occurs within this period. Kuhn states that transition from one paradigm to another occurs when an existing paradigm no longer meets or solves the significant problems effectively. The paradigm gains status and is more successful than its competitors in solving significant problems. Kuhn refers to the transition to a new paradigm as a "scientific revolution." Some authors have expanded on the use of *paradigm* to include a broader world view, often referred to as a *metaparadigm.*

Fawcett (1984) is one author who has defined nursing's metaparadigm as the overall perspective of the nursing discipline. From this perspective, a model for reality and a total view of the discipline are provided. The metaparadigm provides focus for research and theory development within the discipline. According to Fawcett, nursing's metaparadigm, or global perspective, includes the concepts of person, environment, health, and nursing. Within this perspective, paradigms define the concepts of the metaparadigm and serve as a means of organizing observations and guiding methods of study.

Other nursing authors disagree with Fawcett's approach. Hardy (1983) is one nursing author who refers to nursing as being in what Kuhn has referred to as the preparadigm period. She states that until there is agreement on the concepts and one conceptual model of nursing, nursing will not have a metaparadigm. Hardy agrees with most nursing writers that the concepts of person, environment, health, and perhaps nursing are to be considered in the development of conceptual frameworks; however, there is no central agreement on how to view these phenomena.

Newman (1983) has also looked at concepts central to nursing as being the person, environment, and health. She reviewed nursing theorists from Florence Nightingale to present-day theorists within the framework of these central concepts. From this review, Newman concluded that nursing has been generally viewed as being in the preparadigm stage of theory development.

The organization of the concepts within the discipline has been referred to as a *metaparadigm* or *paradigm*, depending on the perspective of the author. Whether the framework for the discipline is referred to as a *metaparadigm* or a *paradigm*, the organization of the concepts forms a world view of the nursing discipline. Some issues relating to the formation of nursing as a discipline include determining which concepts are to be included in giving nursing its unique perspective. For instance, some authors include nursing as a central concept along with person, environment, and health, while others believe that nursing *is* the discipline and cannot be used in defining itself. In this book, the central concepts of nursing are presented as person, environment, and health.

Another issue relating to the formation of nursing as a discipline involves the number of conceptual or theoretical models comprising a discipline. For instance, Watson (1995) and Leininger (1978) believe nursing's conceptualization should involve the concept of care. Newman et al (1991) go so far as to state that if nursing's knowledge does not include caring and human health experiences, it can not be nursing knowledge. Hayne (1992) agrees with others that the unique perspective of nursing is holism or the holistic focus on the concepts of individual, health, and adaptation. Meleis and Trangenstei (1994) believe transition to be a central concept of nursing. Transitions are looked at in relationship to a sense of well-being that is unique to the discipline of nursing. Philips (1995) agrees with the need to study the concepts of nursing as concerned with life processes and evolution rather than specific groups of age, person, or disease. Some authors (e.g., Hardy, 1983) believe that there will be one prevailing model to define nursing, while others (e.g., Fawcett, 1984) believe there are several models. Many current nurse authors (e.g., Moore, 1990; Hayne, 1992) advocate the need for nursing to have more than one theoretical framework in order to advance the discipline. This is called theoretical pluralism and allows for more diversity in thinking and nursing growth. Since nursing is continually evolving and changing, the challenge is to have theories that can respond to new ways of thinking and knowing. The concepts of nursing's paradigm—person, environment, and health—will be discussed in the following sections.

The Concept of Person

The concept of **person** forms the first foundational component of nursing. Individuals are open systems, directly interacting with the internal and external environment. (Systems theory will be discussed in more detail in Chapter 2.) It is important to study the person, various ways of perceiving persons, and their interaction with others. The way we, as individuals and nurses, view or perceive others determines the way we act and interact.

A basic question is, "What is a person?" The person is generally described by a set of attributes or characteristics that are uniquely human. These may be compiled into four major attributes (Anderson, 1974). The first of these four is the capacity to think or to conceptualize on the abstract level. This capacity enables one to stand in the present with a vivid sense of the past and utilize experiences for the future. The capacity to think of oneself in the third person is attributable only to humankind. As a result of this attribute to think or conceptualize, persons are able to use and make tools that help them realize their mental abilities.

This first attribute is closely related to the second, family formation. *Family* may refer to traditional concepts of family or to broader concepts such as social organization (Bruner, 1966). In most instances, the terms *family, culture,* and *social organizations* refer to the interactions of persons joining together to achieve purposes or carry out tasks they could not do individually. Anderson (1974) supports the family as essential for culture development.

A third attribute is the tendency of humans to seek and maintain a territory. Maintenance of territory refers to the establishment of **boundaries** for various social systems and cultures (Anderson, 1974). That is, persons organize in groups with common purposes and establish standards and rules for behavior and patterns of interaction. These standards, rules, and patterns determine the boundaries of the system.

Fourth, humans have the ability to use verbal symbols as language, a means of developing and maintaining culture. It is through transmission of thought that tradition is communicated to future generations. Anderson (1974), in presenting this fourth attribute, hypothesizes that language structures reality. A reality is "more than its vocabulary, grammar, sound structures and so forth; it is also a repository of the modes of thought, the notions of causation and the conceptual and cognitive categories of the culture" (Hymes, 1968, p. 248). Although within recent years many of the Anderson's attributes have been identified in animal cultures, such as language in dolphin populations and complex social structures among many animals, it is the blending of these characteristics in a unique way that continues to identify humans. Dubos (1981) also describes animals as captives of their irreversible biological heritage, whereas humans have the capacity for social evolution, which is reversible and creative. Reilly and Oermann (1992) describe humans as goal directed with continual interaction with the environment. They have mental processes that enable them to think, be creative, organize ideas, and to discriminate and make choices. Each person lives in a private world and seeks balance between thoughts and feelings and the outer world where individuals interact with each other. Several other philosophical approaches to the study of humans will be considered next.

For centuries, people have used a **philosophical approach** that classifies basic natures into two dichotomous categories, good and evil. The idea of the conflict of good and evil is still prevalent in American culture, as reflected in books, cartoons, and television programs. Most of the current literary and philosophical writers recognize that people are neither completely good nor completely evil but contain elements of both. Thus, the search continues for another frame of reference by which to classify human nature.

Researchers have tried to discover that part of humans that makes them unique. They have looked at the biophysical, psychosocial, cultural, and spiritual aspects of the person to discover human nature. Philosophy approaches human nature from an abstract perspective that involves the integration of beliefs and values. How a health care provider perceives and defines the person will be reflected in the type of care rendered. For instance, if the nurse believes that a person is static and unchanging, there will be a tendency not to involve the client in mutual goal setting, whereas a nurse whose philosophy is based on the belief that a person can change is more likely to involve the person in goal setting.

A systems approach views the individual philosophically as more than the sum of parts. Humans are described as open systems. This means that even though they are enclosed within physical bodies, they are not closed off from the **environment.** See Chapter 2 for further discussion on systems theory. Persons are in constant interaction with their surroundings and with others. This interaction creates a continuous exchange of information and knowledge that results in a change within the person, the environment, and others in the environment. An individual's uniqueness lies in the reaction, response, and interaction with the environment, and the individual's concept of self in that environment. Persons are unique, changing, continuous flows of energy with unique needs, ideas, dreams, and goals.

Holistic health has arisen from the philosophical concept of holism introduced by Jan Christian Smuts (1926). It involves the recognition of the whole person within the environment and is consistent with a systems approach. It emphasizes health promotion as well as the treatment of illness. Illness is viewed as an opportunity for growth and a means for developing new strengths within the individual. The holistic perspective recognizes a harmony of people and nature while incorporating the concepts of Eastern and Western health practices. The person's life situation is viewed in terms of individual health practices, such as type and amount of exercise, stress management practices, relationships with others, and avoidance of illness risk factors. Any disruption in an individual's health results in the integration of one of the many methods to restore health.

Some of the methods employed in holistic health practices are meditation, relaxation techniques, medications, biofeedback, nutrition, acupuncture, exercise, surgery, and lifestyle changes. Self-responsibility for health, personal growth, and personal change is basic to the holistic approach in health care. The nurse's responsibility in this approach is to assist the client in identifying the individual strengths and alternatives for health lifestyles.

Clyde Kluckhohn (1953), an anthropologist, presents another approach describing humans in three facets. One facet includes those characteristics shared with all persons, another includes those characteristics shared with some persons, and a third includes those characteristics shared with no one else.

Characteristics shared with all persons involve biological heritage. This entails the physical and psychological growth and developmental stages that all humans experience. Humans grow and function according to their genetic endowment and potential for development in relation to and interaction with their environment.

Kluckhohn's second facet includes those elements shared with some humans. These include social and cultural heritage (e.g., Jewish, Italian, Scandinavian, Irish) and spiritual factors such as seeking life's meaning and one's relationship with the universe.

The third facet identified by Kluckhohn incorporates those characteristics shared with no other person. It includes internal environment, thoughts, ideas, feelings, emotions, values, and beliefs. All of these are conditioned by genetic, social, environmental, cultural, and spiritual background, past experiences, and interactions with others as well as one's response to these. It is this integration and response that make an individual unique.

Abraham Maslow (1943) has identified the person's humanness in terms of a hierarchy of basic needs. He states that needs must be met at the lower levels before the person can invest energy toward meeting needs at higher levels. The meeting of these needs and the desire to satisfy higher needs serve as motivators for human growth. The first level of needs identified by Maslow includes the physiological ones necessary for survival. These include oxygen, food, clothing, sex, rest, comfort, movement, and shelter. Safety and security are the second level. These involve psychological and physical aspects that include continuity, predictability, familiarity, and protection of personal welfare.

The third level, love and belonging, involves intimate, one-to-one relationships, and social or peer group belonging. Some characteristics of this level are affection, closeness, support, reassurance. and affiliation. The fourth level, self-esteem, embraces a sense of self-worth, dignity, privacy, approval, respect and self-reliance.

Self-actualization is the highest level of Maslow's hierarchy. This concerns the recognition and realization of individual potential and innate capabilities. It has to do with the individual's feelings of satisfaction with oneself and one's life. Maslow believes that humans continually strive to reach and maintain self-actualization and work through these levels in order to meet this goal. He thinks that few persons ever reach this final level.

As a person's environment, internal systems, and responses change, the person changes. An individual is not stagnant but continually changing, growing, and responding to changes and growth. Therefore, humans are said to be dynamic beings, continually adapting to maintain homeodynamics, or a relative balance within themselves and their environment.

This changing and growing has been termed by **Carl Rogers** as "becoming." It involves "a person who is learning to live his life as a participant in a fluid, ongoing process, in which he is continually discovering new aspects of himself in the flow of his experience" (1961, p. 124) and entails the process of becoming totally human.

Rogers has listed directions his clients have taken in the process of becoming totally human. These are: move away from facades, give up being what one is not; move away from "oughts," away from doing what one should only because it is what one "should" do; away from meeting the expectations of others and from trying always to please others. He sees the person as moving toward self direction; toward the "being process," becoming aware of one's own dynamic, changing self; toward complexity, looking at things not just as black and white or good and bad, but as interrelated and integrated; toward openness to experience, being aware of one's own feelings, and being able to take risks and be close, develop trust, and be free to experience new things and feelings; toward acceptance of others as they are, and toward trust of oneself and one's capabilities, so that one may value self and feelings.

These writers have attempted to discover the uniqueness of humankind. Figure 1–1 summarizes the various philosophical approaches to the study of the person. It is important for each of us to identify and develop a personal philosophy. This can help in the integration of values and beliefs and will influence our approach to persons in giving nursing care. Viewing humans as unique growing, dynamic beings, whose whole comprises more than the sum of the parts and who are in constant interaction with the environment and others in the environment, provides some parameters for developing a philosophy of humankind. Persons, unique and interacting provide the basis and major focus of nursing.

Nursing theorists have developed the concept of the person in the development of theories. Some of the ideas central to their view of the person are presented in Chapter 2. This chapter continues with separate discussions of the environment and health. These concepts are then developed as they interface with one another to become part of the foundations of nursing.

The Concept of Environment

The dictionary defines *environment* as "the aggregate of external circumstances, conditions, and things that affect the existence and development of an individual, organism, or group." The concept of environment in nursing is more encompassing than this definition. There is an internal environment that includes a person's thoughts, abilities, self-concept, physical and chemical makeup, ambitions, and spiritual and psychosocial essence. An external environment consists of physical surroundings, interaction with other persons, social systems, community, country, and universe.

The external and internal environments of the person are in continual interaction and energy exchange. The person responds to changes within the environment as the environment responds to and exchanges energy within the person. Since this is an internal and external exchange, it becomes impossible to separate the environment from the person. Change is effected, and responses are made to these changes. Thus, the person and environment are considered open systems, and the interaction of these is considered to be an open exchange of energy.

APPROACH	DIAGRAM OF THE APPROACH	DESCRIPTION OF THE APPROACH
GOOD-EVIL	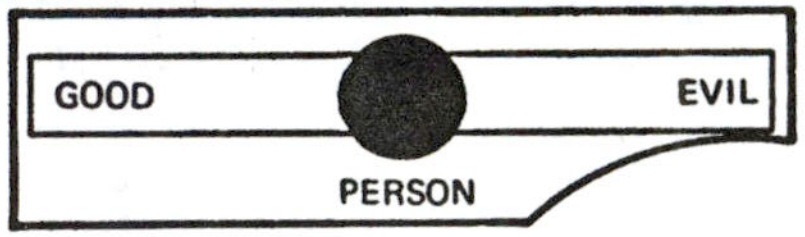	The person's nature can be classified as basically good or evil.
SYSTEMS	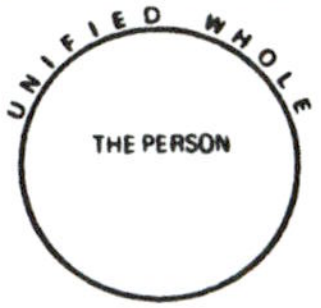	Persons are open systems, more than the sum of their parts, and are in constant interaction with their surroundings and others. Persons are unique, changing, continuous flows of energy. (von Bertalanffy)
SHARED CHARACTERISTICS	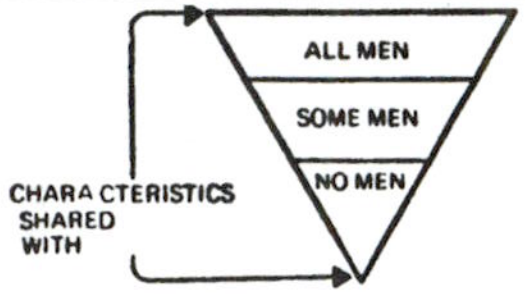	Describes persons in three facets; those characteristics shared with all, those characteristics shared with some, and those characteristics shared with no one. The characteristics shared with no one contribute to the person's uniqueness. (Kluckhohn)
HUMAN NEEDS	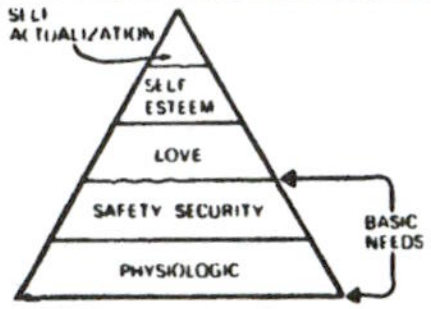	The person's humanness is identified in terms of a hierarchy of needs. Lower-level needs must be met before energy can be directed toward higher-level needs. Persons strive to reach and maintain self-actualization. (Maslow)
BECOMING PROCESS	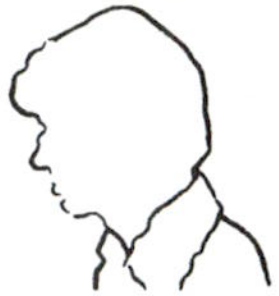	Persons are continually changing, growing, and responding to change and growth. They are adapting and discovering new aspects of themselves in the process of "becoming totally human." (Rogers)

Figure 1–1. Summary of the philosophical approaches to the study of the person.

One of the components of environment that has influenced the person and health care is **society.** Society represents a structure of the relationships between persons. It can be defined as a group of people who regularly interact with one another and have common goals. The dynamic interaction can occur among individuals, families, and communities. In Kluckhohn's conception, society represents a part of those characteristics that people share with some others. Through society, **culture** (the way of life of the people) is manifested. The way of looking at life is reflected through values and beliefs developed by a people. For example, democracy and freedom are cultural values developed early in American history and reflect shared ideas concerning the nature of humans and their social life. Culture includes social standards with norms and rules that define certain acceptable and nonacceptable behaviors, which are transmitted to others. Foods, rituals, and language customs are clues to the culture of a particular group.

Norms, rules, and laws are found in every society. *Norms* are standards containing some degree of morality, whereas *rules* do not have moral implications. Norms and rules may be mere practices or may be formalized legally as laws. For example, there are rules and norms in nursing practice, referred to as standards of practice, which are not formalized in law but guide and influence the quality and nature of nurses' practice. In addition, there are Nurse Practice Acts in most states that form legal parameters. Since these parameters differ from state to state, it is important that each practitioner be familiar with the specific practice act in the individual jurisdiction. Other more informal norms in nursing practice might include patterns of interaction with other health care professionals, such as physicians, social workers, and pharmacists.

Culture affects and is affected by dynamic changes, which are happening at a rapid pace in American society. For instance, a trend has been seen in population shifts from rural to urban areas and back to rural areas, thus affecting cultural patterns. A cultural change such as the population mobility affects health care. At a time when there are increased numbers of urban residents, environmental pollution increased and became a major concern because of its effect on respiratory function. As patterns again change, different health problems will become evident. Another example of cultural change is noted in altered attitudes such as the belief that health care is a right, not just a privilege. A third example of the impact of culture on society and health care practices is reflected in the beliefs and perpetuation of old wives' tales, such as applying butter to a burn despite documented evidence of the negative effects. Each societal change includes the types and patterns of disease and related health practices. The environment, though named as a primary concept for

nursing, does not always gain the prominence needed. It is not sufficient in today's world to focus only on change in individuals as they
interact with the environment, but there is a major need to also focus
on systemic societal change needed to foster conditions for optimal
health for all persons. As an example, nurses must put pressure on
the political and social systems that will ensure administration of
services for quality health care of our increased aging population.

Nursing theorists have presented differing views of the environment and its relation to person, health, and nursing. Martha
Rogers (1970) describes the environment as being continuous with
the person, in constant energy exchange, and without boundaries.
King (1981) conceptualizes the environment as having internal and
external elements involving temporal and spatial reality. Roy & Andrews (1991) discuss environment as conditions, circumstances, and
surrounding influences that affect the individual.

The Concept of Health

The third component of the foundation of nursing is the concept of
health. **Health** is defined and influenced by the interactive forces of
environment with individuals or groups. These forces may interact
functionally or dysfunctionally, producing varying states of health.
Nursing came into existence to effect a positive direction on health.
Whether it is primary (prevention), secondary (treatment), or tertiary (rehabilitation), nursing plays a major part in health care.

Over the years, several definitions of health have appeared in
the literature. The United Nations World Health Organization defines health as "a state of complete physical, mental, and social well-
being and not merely the absence of disease or infirmity" (World
Health Organization, 1974). Health can also be defined simply as
having a sound body and mind. Consider these questions: What is
health? Does it involve daily exercise, a balanced diet, regular physical exams, or "good clean living"? Is health the absence of illness or
is it merely a person's perception of his or her state of health?

Other definitions of health include "the state of optimum capacity of an individual for the effective performance of his roles and
tasks" (Parsons, 1959). Thus, Parsons' definition of health is in terms
of role. Individuals may assume many roles during life. When a person feels good, a health role is assumed. A person who feels ill may
take on the sick role. Parsons defined four aspects of the sick role.
The first aspect is that the person is not held responsible for illness.
The second aspect is that the person is exempt from usual social
tasks. For example, when an individual has a viral infection, absence
from work is permissible. The third aspect of the sick role is that the

individual has the obligation to become well. It is not socially acceptable to be ill for an extended period of time. With this approach, persons with chronic illnesses such as emphysema, alcoholism, or arthritis may have difficulty being accepted because of society's intolerance of prolonged illness. The fourth aspect is that the individual must seek competent help to treat the illness. According to this approach, although the illness is socially acceptable, the person has the responsibility to take action that will alleviate the condition. Every individual assumes the sick role in a unique manner.

Dunn (1959a, 1959b) defined health as the opposite of illness. He views health on a continuum influenced by many environmental factors. No person has either absolute health or absolute illness but is on a continuum from peak wellness at one extreme to illness and death at the other. The areas in between these extreme points include serious illness, minor illness, and freedom from illness.

High-level wellness has been defined as functioning at one's best. It means that the potential of the individual is maximized and utilized within the individual's environment (Dunn, 1959a, 1959b). In this approach, a person who has a paralysis of a leg would be considered healthy if able to carry out tasks within optimum capacity. When the goal of health care is high-level wellness, health care practitioners are committed to assisting individuals to maximize their potential within their environment. This last part, "within their environment," has become the focus of some new ways of looking at health care and the delivery of services.

As one can see from the many definitions of health, no one definition is ideal; all have major limitations. The important idea to abstract from these definitions is that health is dynamic and ever changing, not a stagnant state. Health can be measured only in relative terms. No one is absolutely healthy or ill. In addition, health applies to the total person, including progression toward the realization and fulfillment of one's potential as well as maintaining physical, psychosocial health.

Nurses have defined health in terms of their theories of nursing. Health has been identified as wholeness and integrity (Orem, 1991) or as adjustments to stressors in daily living (King, 1981). Current nursing theory conferences have presented new thoughts on health which suggest that health may not best be defined in terms of a continuum. Some theorists suggest that individuals define health from their own perspective.

Because health is an ambiguous term, nurse authors such as Leininger (1978), Fawcet (1984), and Meleis (1994) argue that the focus of nursing should be on the concept of well-being and not on health as such. They argue that this helps escape from the concept of the disease model of medicine and that it better explains the phenomena of interest to nursing.

INFLUENCES ON HEALTH

Many factors influence health, such as social values, age, sex, education, socioeconomic status, religion, culture, and attitudes. This section focuses on some of the influences on the health of persons. The influences to be discussed include the consumer movement, health benefits, technological advances, financing of health care, population shifts and lifestyles, and stress.

The Consumer Movement

One of the most current influences is the impact of the **consumer movement** on health. The general public continues to become more aware of the need to participate actively in health care.

During the 1960s, the concept of the patient as a consumer came into being. This applied a market concept to the field of health. In this context, the client is viewed as a consumer, purchasing service—in this case, health service. In consumer–provider relationships, the consumer has considerably more bargaining power than formerly and may even be able to shop in the marketplace of health care. Thus, the use of the term *consumer* to replace *client* or *patient* initiated a different perspective and changed the relationship between health care providers and clients.

The consumer influence has become most prominent in the past few years with the skyrocketing cost of health care. People have an increased need for information and knowledge. No longer is the carte blanche "to do whatever is needed" acceptable, and informed consent is a must for the health consumer.

Other rights have emerged as a result of this societal consumer movement. The consumer is no longer content to follow the advice of health care providers blindly. Consumers are beginning to exert pressure for what is considered to be their right to high-quality health care and are demanding to receive it at an affordable price. Other societal factors that have energized the consumer movement include more consumer protection agencies in government, initiated legislative actions, improved health care mandated by labor unions for workers, more health education for consumers, and increased use of the media to publicize health issues. In addition, in 1992, the American Hospital Association revised a **Patient's Bill of Rights** to inform consumers, primarily hospitalized patients, of their entitled rights relative to health care. This bill of rights is as follows:

A PATIENT'S BILL OF RIGHTS

Introduction

Effective health care requires collaboration between patients and physicians and other health care professionals. Open and honest communication, respect for personal and professional values, and sensitivity to differences are integral to optimal patient care. As the setting for the provision of health services, hospitals must provide a foundation for understanding and respecting the rights and responsibilities of patients, their families, physicians, and other caregivers. Hospitals must ensure a health care ethic that respects the role of patients in decision making about treatment choices and other aspects of their care. Hospitals must be sensitive to cultural, racial, linguistic, religious, age, gender, and other differences as well as the needs of persons with disabilities.

The American Hospital Association presents *A Patient's Bill of Rights* with the expectation that it will contribute to more effective patient care and be supported by the hospital on behalf of the institution, its medical staff, employees, and patients. The American Hospital Association encourages health care institutions to tailor this bill of rights to their patient community by translating and/or simplifying the language of this bill of rights as may be necessary to ensure that patients and their families understand their rights and responsibilities.

Bill of Rights*

1. The patient has the right to considerate and respectful care.
2. The patient has the right to and is encouraged to obtain from physicians and other direct caregivers relevant, current, and understandable information concerning diagnosis, treatment, and prognosis.

   Except in emergencies when the patient lacks decision-making capacity and the need for treatment is urgent, the patient is entitled to the opportunity to discuss and request information related to the specific procedures and/or treatments, the risks involved, the possible length of recuperation, and the medically reasonable alternatives and their accompanying risks and benefits.

   Patients have the right to know the identity of physicians, nurses, and others involved in their care, as well as when

---

*These rights can be exercised on the patient's behalf by a designated surrogate or proxy decision maker if the patient lacks decision-making capacity, is legally incompetent, or is a minor.

those involved are students, residents, or other trainees. The patient also has the right to know the immediate and long-term financial implications of treatment choices, insofar as they are known.

3. The patient has the right to make decisions about the plan of care prior to and during the course of treatment and to refuse a recommended treatment or plan of care to the extent permitted by law and hospital policy and to be informed of the medical consequences of this action. In case of such refusal, the patient is entitled to other appropriate care and services that the hospital provides or transfer to another hospital. The hospital should notify patients of any policy that might affect patient choice within the institution.

4. The patient has the right to have an advance directive (such as a living will, health care proxy, or durable power of attorney for health care) concerning treatment or designating a surrogate decision maker with the expectation that the hospital will honor the intent of that directive to the extent permitted by law and hospital policy.

   Health care institutions must advise patients of their rights under state law and hospital policy to make informed medical choices, ask if the patient has an advance directive, and include that information in patient records. The patient has the right to timely information about hospital policy that may limit its ability to implement fully a legally valid advance directive.

5. The patient has the right to every consideration of privacy. Case discussion, consultation, examination, and treatment should be conducted so as to protect each patient's privacy.

6. The patient has the right to expect that all communications and records pertaining to his/her care will be treated as confidential by the hospital, except in cases such as suspected abuse and public health hazards when reporting is permitted or required by law. The patient has the right to expect that the hospital will emphasize the confidentiality of this information when it releases it to any other parties entitled to review information in these records.

7. The patient has the right to review the records pertaining to his/her medical care and to have the information explained or interpreted as necessary, except when restricted by law.

8. The patient has the right to expect that, within its capacity and policies, a hospital will make reasonable response to the request of a patient for appropriate and medically indicated care and services. The hospital must provide evaluation, service, and/or referral as indicated by the urgency of

the case. When medically appropriate and legally permissible, or when a patient has so requested, a patient may be transferred to another facility. The institution to which the patient is to be transferred must first have accepted the patient for transfer. The patient must also have the benefit of complete information and explanation concerning the need for, risks, benefits, and alternatives to such a transfer.

9. The patient has the right to ask and be informed of the existence of business relationships among the hospital, educational institutions, other health care providers, or payers that may influence the patient's treatment and care.

10. The patient has the right to consent to or decline to participate in proposed research studies or human experimentation affecting care and treatment or requiring direct patient involvement, and to have those studies fully explained prior to consent. A patient who declines to participate in research or experimentation is entitled to the most effective care that the hospital can otherwise provide.

11. The patient has the right to expect reasonable continuity of care when appropriate and to be informed by physicians and other caregivers of available and realistic patient care options when hospital care is no longer appropriate.

12. The patient has the right to be informed of hospital policies and practices that relate to patient care, treatment and responsibilities. The patient has the right to be informed of available resources for resolving disputes, grievances, and conflicts, such as ethics committees, patient representatives, or other mechanisms available in the institution. The patient has the right to be informed of the hospital's charges for services and available payment methods.

The collaborative nature of health care requires that patients, or their families/surrogates, participate in their care. The effectiveness of care and patient satisfaction with the course of treatment depend, in part, on the patient fulfilling certain responsibilities. Patients are responsible for providing information about past illnesses, hospitalizations, medications, and other matters related to health status. To participate effectively in decision making, patients must be encouraged to take responsibility for requesting additional information or clarification about their health status or treatment when they do not fully understand information and instructions. Patients are also responsible for ensuring that the health care institution has a copy of their written advance directive if they have one. Patients are responsible for informing their physicians and other caregivers if they anticipate problems in following prescribed treatment.

Patients should also be aware of the hospital's obligation to be reasonably efficient and equitable in providing care to other patients and the community. The hospital's rules and regulations are designed to help the hospital meet this obligation. Patients and their families are responsible for making reasonable accommodations to the needs of the hospital, other patients, medical staff, and hospital employees. Patients are responsible for providing necessary information for insurance claims and for working with the hospital to make payment arrangements, when necessary.

A person's health depends on much more than health care services. Patients are responsible for recognizing the impact of their lifestyle on their personal health.

Conclusion

Hospitals have many functions to perform, including the enhancement of health status, health promotion, and the prevention and treatment of injury and disease; the immediate and ongoing care and rehabilitation of patients; the education of health professionals, patients, and the community; and research. All these activities must be conducted with an overriding concern for the values and dignity of patients.

(Reprinted with the permission of the American Hospital Association; copyright © 1992.)

The consumer movement not only has influenced the client as a consumer but also has resulted in some societal trends for health care. One trend is allowing the client a choice in health care and more direct involvement in health planning, whether it is planning for personal health care or serving on community, state, or other health boards. Provision for comprehensive care, as well as preventative services, is a second trend. A third resultant trend is protecting the natural environment essential to life. Fourth, society continues to identify ways by which persons may have access to a broad range of information on health, illness, disability, and ways in which individuals can protect and improve their personal health.

The consumer movement led to the passage of the National Consumer Health Information and Health Promotion Act of 1976, which provides for a national program of health information, promotion, preventive health services, and education in the appropriate use of health care. An Office of Health information and Health Promotion was established within the Office of the Assistant Secretary for Health. The introduction of the consumer movement into the health care system has resulted in the fifth trend, a change in health care from curative to preventive care.

Not all of the changes in consumer health care have been positive. For example, there was a rapid and substantial fall in the death rate for all age groups in the first half of the 20th century. However, there has been an increase in death rates from chronic disease along with exceptionally high infant death rates in the urban ghettoes. These infant deaths have often occurred within a few miles of clinical facilities. Recent econometric studies have found that the environmental variables, especially income and education, are far more important determinants of death rates than the availability of medical care. This underscores the relationships of health conditions to environmental and socioeconomic problems and the impossibility of correcting health deficiencies solely through improved medical care.

Health Beliefs

Related to the consumer movement is the concept of health belief and health behavior. A model of health belief was presented by Rosenstock (1966) as an explanation of determinants of health behavior and of preventive health behavior. The model and subsequent adaptations of it have been used as a perspective for examining factors influencing client behaviors on behalf of their own or significant others' health. Barriers to health care may include objective health behaviors related to physical proximity and availability of transportation to health care services, as well as subjective barriers related to client perceptions of their health. Client health beliefs and perceptions and consequent health behaviors are significant influences on client health.

Technological Advances

Major advances in technology also influence health. Technology, as well as providing benefits in diagnosis and treatment, has created challenges. Fragmentation of care has occurred as a result of the increased numbers of health care workers required by advanced technology and consequent specialization. An individual in the hospital may see as many as 20 to 30 health care providers. Educational cost to train new personnel in the knowledge and skills of specialization are resulting in increased cost to the consumer. Complex equipment has also increased cost factors. Obsolescence of expensive health equipment continually pushes up the cost as newer models become available. The diagnostic tool magnetic resonance imaging (MRI) is an example of machinery that has led to increased cost. To facilitate the use of the MRI for total populations, many hospitals have grouped together to purchase and share the unit, thus decreasing the expense.

Financing Health Care

As a result of these and other technological advances, financing health care is a primary concern of every consumer, since the cost of even a short period of hospitalization could be financially crippling. Several methods have developed for financing rising health costs. One of the more common methods is through private for profit companies such as Columbia-CSA-HS or membership in a health maintenance organization such as Kaiser Permanente. Other common methods are public insurances such as Medicare and Medicaid, which are available to the elderly and other qualified individuals. Industry and business may offer insurance plans for employees as a benefit to help with health care costs.

Because the cost of a day's hospitalization has increased as much as 30 times since the early 1900s, more emphasis is being placed on prevention of illness. Preventive treatment is classified in three areas: primary prevention, or promoting health and preventing disease; secondary prevention, or early detection of health care problems; and tertiary prevention, or the prompt and continual rehabilitation after an illness. Some of the health maintenance programs aimed at the preventive treatment described include maternal child health programs; mental health programs; and environmental, nutritional, and dental health programs. Prevention programs focus on health problems such as hypertension, safety, and pollution. Each preventive program has a cost factor that is ultimately assumed by the consumer.

The development of **diagnosis-related group (DRG)** categories for establishing billing categories for U.S. hospitals reimbursed by Medicare as a health cost containment measure has had a significant impact on the provision of nursing care. Payment is based on predetermined costs related to the treatment of the specific medical diagnosis of the hospitalized client. Initially, 383 categories were identified and arranged in a hierarchy. The payments are made on estimated costs for a hospitalized patient given the medical diagnosis. Hospitals profit when the length of hospitalization is shorter than projected and experience loss when costs exceed the established standard. This payment plan is an attempt to decrease unnecessary testing and hospitalization of clients. An extension of the DRG for billing is the resource utilization group (RUG) for in-patient long-term care. These types of systems do not take into account needed nursing as identified through nursing diagnosis and therefore influence nursing services that can be provided.

Health care is no longer institutionally based. It is becoming more and more community-based. Nursing care in the community started in the early 1900s; by the year 2010, 70 percent of nursing care will occur in the home. Thus, nursing needs a theory base that focuses on health promotion, environment, and the quality of life (Clarke & Cody, 1994).

Population Shifts and Life-Styles

Another influence on health is the increased population. With an increase in life expectancy, there has been an increase in the number of the elderly in our country. Today, there are 37.1 million Americans over 60, and the U.S. Bureau of the Census estimates that there will be 40 million by the year 2000, the majority of whom will be women. Thus, the field of gerontology is a rapidly growing specialty. People are living longer with a subsequent increase in chronic illness.

Uneven distribution of health care facilities and resources has been especially detrimental to rural areas and inner cities. One geographic area may have a larger number of highly competent health care providers, while another may have few or none. The mobility and change of the American population cause special problems in health care delivery. Rarely does one physician or nurse know a patient from birth through adulthood. Therefore, health care professionals rely more on health histories from the client than on past health records for gathering information to assist in client care. Mobility has also affected health personnel. Health care professionals may not practice in the area where they grew up and, therefore, may not be familiar with the special health concerns and needs unique to the area and population.

People's lifestyles often do not promote health. Some reasons for this may be a limited appreciation of the effect of lifestyle on health, difficulty accepting responsibility for personal health, lack of knowledge, decrease in economic resources, denial of disease and death, and varying perceptions of consumer health.

Lifestyles and occupations create unique health care problems. For example, stress in American society has contributed to increased incidence of physical and psychological illnesses. In addition, the identification of acquired immune deficiency syndrome (AIDS) among IV-drug users and persons with unprotected sexual encounters has focused attention on other lifestyles that present health risks. Occupational factors have increased the incidence of black lung disease among coal miners, a condition unique to that population.

Our society has also witnessed the revolution of rising expectations. More informed attitudes about health and greater financial support for health care have increased demand for all health services. People want energy, vitality, even perpetual youth and beauty. Artificial organs, organ transplants, cosmetic surgery, and pacemakers are examples of advances that maintain and enhance our lives. However, the discrepancy between the rate of expenditure for health and the improvement in health status appears to be increasing. Moreover, mortality figures in the United States reflect the population's excessive intake of animal protein, fats, alcohol, tobacco, and drugs.

Stress

Health is influenced by and is dependent on the degree and amount of **stress**, as well as the perception of it by the individual. It is conceptualized within a particular theoretical approach. For example, from an adaptive response perspective, stress may occur when a person's adaptive responses are inadequate for the situation. Persons strive for homeodynamics, and stress results when the individual experiences fear of the unknown or perceives a threatened loss. Stress has been viewed as both psychological and physical. Both types of stress result in changes in an individual's state of health when the coping mechanisms employed to reduce the stress level are no longer sufficient. Selye (1956) defined stress as a "nonspecific response of the body to any demand made upon it." Stressors may be either positive or negative, but repeated exposures over time can lead to physical aging and ultimately death. Many diseases have been related to stress. Stressors can be physical, psychological, cultural, or social. They are factors that put a strain on the person. Stress affects each person in a different manner, and the individual's reactions and adaptation to stress are unique.

Selye has described stress and the body's response to it as the general adaptation syndrome (GAS). This syndrome consists of three stages: (1) *alarm stage*, which is the initial physiological response to any stress and consists of chemical and hormonal changes to prepare the body to meet the stress; (2) *stage of resistance*, which involves the changes necessary for the body's fight to maintain a balance or homeostasis; and (3) *stage of exhaustion*, which occurs if the body is unable to maintain a homeostatic balance and results in the loss of the body's ability to adapt. If uninterrupted, this stage will continue until death. Stress is not an emotion or feeling but a response or syndrome produced by the body in adapting to some external or internal factor. It is an individual's adjustive response to an unmet need.

Lazarus (1966) describes psychological stress. He identifies psychological stress as concerning "the meaning or significance of a stimulus, that is, its capacity to produce harm that has not yet occurred" (p. 424). Physiological stress "concerns harm or disturbances of the tissue structure or function that has already occurred" (p. 424).

Lazarus describes four classes of reactions that have been typically used to index stress. These are (1) reports of disturbed affects such as fear, anger, and depression; (2) motor–behavioral reactions such as tremors, increased muscle tone, and facial expressions, and fight or flight; (3) changes in the adequacy of cognitive functioning (facilitation or impairment); and (4) physiological changes involving hormonal, chemical, and nervous systems. *Coping* is identified by Lazarus as the strategies used for dealing with threat. He discusses primary threat appraisal and secondary or cognitive appraisal. Secondary appraisal intervenes between the threat and the coping process to help choose the appropriate coping form.

From a systems perspective, stimuli to a system can be considered as potential stressors. Potential stressors may challenge the system in a positive or negative way. The boundaries of the system screen stressors. Reverberation results from stressor stimulations (Joos et al., 1985).

Stress has been studied by many disciplines. The identification of the term within a nursing framework adds to the ability of nurses to utilize the concept in research, theory, and knowledge development. Dr. Imogene King (1981) and Sr. Callista Roy (1991) are two nurse theorists who have conceptualized stress within a nursing perspective. Stress is defined by King as "a dynamic state whereby a human being interacts with the environment to maintain balance for growth, development, and performance, which involves an exchange of energy and information between the person and the environment for regulation and control of stressors" (King, 1981, p. 98). Stress is viewed as an essential concept in understanding the interpersonal system. King describes several means to reduce stress in nursing situations, such as listening to and talking with the individual; giving adequate explanations of procedures, tests, and treatments; helping to understand events occurring in the health care setting; and involving family members in the care of the individual.

Roy conceptualizes stress as adaptation. She defines stress as "the general term given to the transaction between the environment demand for adaptation and the person's response" (Roy & Roberts, 1981, p. 54). Stressors are described as focal stimuli that are mediated by contextual and residual factors to produce, in part, the interaction called stress. The other half of stress is described as coping mechanisms, which, when activated, produce adaptive or ineffective responses. The stressors may be physical, physiological, psychosocial, or a combination of these. The coping mechanisms are described as "any attempt to master a new situation that can be potentially threatening, frustrating, challenging, or gratifying" (Roy & Roberts, 1981, p. 56).

RELATIONSHIP OF PERSON, ENVIRONMENT, AND HEALTH TO NURSING

When people need help promoting and maintaining their health, dealing with illness, obtaining rehabilitation assistance, or dealing with problems relating to their definitions of health and illness, they turn to "experts" or "professionals" in the health care fields. People needed and sought assistance for health long before nursing became a profession or an organized occupation. Traditionally, assistance in meeting daily physical needs has been associated with nursing. Emphasis in nursing is being given to helping people with the difficulties they are experiencing in daily living. Therefore, nurses can promote health in any context in which a person lives. The nurse serves as a "translator" between social systems, attempting to understand the culture and health beliefs of the person requiring or seeking assistance. Nurses have an interdependent role with other health care professionals in the treatment of a disability or illness. They also have a primary role in helping the person live with or avoid further disability, improving wellness, and living to the fullest capabilities.

Nursing's focus has been on quality of human life at a time when society was mainly concerned with basic biological survival. Thus, "quality of human life" has lacked societal significance and, as a result, nursing has not been generally valued by society. Nursing has in large part focused on the individual client and family and in general, as reported by observers of the effects of society and the environment on people, collective energy has not been directed to effecting systemic change. Think for a moment of homelessness in American society and the consequent devastation of poverty, poor nutrition, loss of meaning and dignity in life often experienced by those who are homeless. Nursing today calls for nurses to expand their energies beyond the individual within the immediate surroundings toward influencing the structures that influence health and nursing.

Nursing is no longer solely cure-oriented but focuses on health-seeking behaviors of individuals. Nurses have both independent and collaborative roles with other members of the health care team. As the present trend in the delivery of health care services continues to be away from the hospital and back into the community, nurses are becoming increasingly aware of their potential to influence health and provide affordable quality care. Nurses must critically analyze the impact of factors such as changing health care reimbursement systems like the DRG system as they relate to the provision of quality nursing care.

The person is in constant, continuous interaction with the environment in an attempt to promote, improve, and maintain health. An individual's health is affected by environmental conditions. The person's internal and external environments also influence the health of that individual. Disturbances in environmental factors lead to disturbances in the health of the individual. When the disturbances become too stressful to compensate for, persons may see a change in their health status.

Figure 1–2 illustrates the interrelationship of the components of theory, practice, and research to the concepts of person, environment, health, and nursing as foundations of the discipline of nursing.

The discipline of nursing may be thought of as an open system maintained in dynamic equilibrium through constant input, feedback, and the systematic interaction of theory, research, and practice. Using systems theory as an approach to nursing has several advantages. First, it allows us to view individuals and the environment in terms of the many factors that interact to influence health. Second, it links many theories and concepts into a meaningful framework by which decisions can be made. Third, it provides a common language for numerous disciplines, each having its own body of knowledge and area of specialization. Shared meanings provide a basis for interaction in conceptualization of common goals in health care. For example, a psychologist may focus primarily on the psychological aspects of the person, while a sociologist may focus on the sociocultural aspects of the person. In the systems approach, all disciplines view the person as a whole, with all aspects interacting together. Finally, the approach is dynamic, with change and growth as ongoing parts of the life process. This approach allows the nurse to interact with clients with respect for their complexity and capacity for change.

However, the systems approach to care, cause and effect relationships, and ways of knowing is being discussed as antiquated in view of changing world view. Watson (1995) describes the evolving concept of **postmodernism** in the development of nursing knowledge. She states that in this period of changing centuries, there is both the beginning and the end of modernity. The dominance of the Western world view of one reality and linear thinking is ending, allowing for the understanding of many realities. This questions the approach to knowledge development as a scientific endeavor, which controls and dominates the world, to explain and describe reality by the equation knowledge equals science, which equals reality. Nurses must be ready to challenge themselves and their ideas to develop means of understanding and helping individuals using multiple theories and ways of knowing.

Paradoxically, the health care system today, which includes nursing, is characterized by the tension of impending change. Factors contributing to this change relate to views of society regarding health that perpetuate trends away from an illness orientation to a health promotion and maintenance orientation. The process of adjusting and adapting to change becomes a major focus of health care delivery.

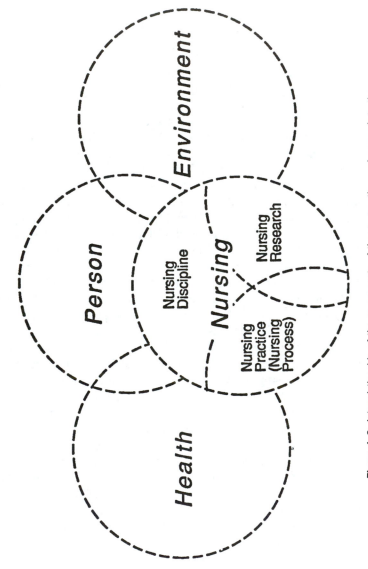

Figure 1–2. Interrelationship of the components of theory, practice, and research to the concepts of person, environment, health, and nursing as foundations of the discipline of nursing.

SUMMARY

Nursing as a discipline has been defined and has been conceptualized in terms of the foundations or central concepts of nursing: person, environment, and health. The focus of nursing is the dynamic interaction of others within their environment. Individuals are not isolated but exist in environments with fellow human beings. Health is being redefined continually. The health status of the American people reflects the impact of the demographic, socioeconomic, and cultural trends of our nation. Nursing has grown and is changing in response to these trends and the changing needs of persons in society.

▶ Questions for Discussion

1. How would you describe the discipline of nursing?
2. Differentiate between the view points of a paradigm.
3. Briefly describe the components of theory, practice, and research as they relate to the discipline of nursing.
4. Name the foundations of the discipline of nursing as outlined in this chapter.
5. What is your philosophy of humankind? How do you see this philosophy influencing your nursing care?
6. What environmental changes can you identify that have influenced health?
7. Formulate a definition of health, using the definitions presented.
8. How does nursing relate to changing definitions of the person, environment, and health?
9. What is your personal opinion of the goodness or badness of the person at birth?
10. Do you believe people are capable of change? Why or why not?

REFERENCES

American Hospital Association. *A Patient's Bill of Rights.* Chicago: The Association; 1992.

American Nurses Association. *Nursing: A Social Policy Statement.* Kansas City, MO: ANA; 1980.

American Nurses Association. *Nursing: A Social Policy Statement.* Washington, DC: American Nurses Publishing; 1995.

Anderson RC. *Human Behavior in the Social Environment.* Chicago: Aldine Publishing; 1974.

Bruner J. *Toward a Theory of Instruction.* Cambridge, MA: Belknap Press; 1966.

Clarke P, Cody W. Nursing theory-based practice in the home and community: The crux of professional nursing education. *Adv Nurs Sci.* 1994; 17(2):41–53.

Dickoff J, Wiedenbach E. Theory in a practice discipline. *Nurs Research.* 1968; 17(5):415–435.

Donaldson S, Crowley D. The discipline of nursing. *Nurs Outlook.* 1978; 26:113–120.

Dubos R. *Celebrations of Life.* New York: McGraw-Hill; 1981.

Dunn H. High-level wellness. *Am J Pub-Health.* 1959a; 49:786.

Dunn H. What high-level wellness means. *Can J Pub Health.* 1959b; 50:447.

Fawcett J. The metaparadigm of nursing: Present status and future refinements. *Image.* 1984; 16(3):84–86.

Glaser B, Strauss A. *Discovery of Grounded Theory. Strategies for Qualitative Research.* Chicago: Aldine Publishing; 1961.

Green JA. Science, nursing, and nursing science: A conceptual analysis. *Adv Nurs Sci,* 1979; 2(1):57–64.

Hardy M. Metaparadigms in theory development. In: Chaska NL, ed. *The Nursing Profession: A Time to Speak.* New York: McGraw-Hill; 1983.

Hayne Y. The current status and future significance of nursing as a discipline. *J Adv Nurs.* 1992; 17:104–107.

Hymes D. Functions of speech: An evolutionary approach. In: Wiehude A, ed. *Man in Adaptation: The Biosocial Background.* Chicago: Aldine Publishing; 1968.

Jacox A. Theory construction in nursing: An overview. *Nurs Res.* 1974; 23: 4-13.

Joos I, Nelson R, Lyness A. *Man, Health, and Nursing: Basic Concepts and Theories.* Reston, VA: Reston Publishing Co; 1985.

King I. *A Theory for Nursing.* New York: Wiley; 1981.

Kluckhohn C. *Personality in Nature, Society and Culture.* New York: Knopf; 1953.

Kuhn TS. *The Nature of Scientific Revolution.* 2nd ed. Chicago: University of Chicago Press; 1970.

Lazarus RS. *Psychological Stress and the Coping Process.* New York: McGraw-Hill; 1966.

Leninger M. *Transcultural Nursing: Concepts, Theories, and Practices.* New York: Wiley; 1978.

Maslow AA. A theory of human motivation. *Psychol Rev.* 1943; 50:370–396.

Meleis A, Trangenstein P. Facilitating transitions: Redefinition of the nursing mission. *Nurs Outlook.* 1994; 42:255–259.

Merton R. On sociological theories of the middle range. In: *On Theoretical Sociology.* New York: The Free Press; 1977.

Moore S. Thoughts on the discipline of nursing as we approach the year 2000. *J Adv Nurs.* 1990; 15:825–828.

Newman M, Sime A, Corcoran-Perry S. The focus of the discipline of nursing. *Adv Nurs Sci.* 1991; 14(1):1–6.

Newman MA. The continuing revolution: A history of nursing science. In: Chasta N, ed. *The Nursing Profession: A Time to Speak.* New York: McGraw-Hill; 1983.

Orem DE. *Nursing: Concepts of Practice.* 4th ed. St. Louis: Mosby Year Book; 1991.

Parsons T. Definitions of health and illness in the light of American values and social structure. In: Jaco E, ed. *Patients, Physicians and Illness.* Glencoe, NY: The Free Press; 1959.

Philips Jr. Nursing theory-based research for advanced nursing practice. *Nurs Sci Q.* 8; 1:4–5.

Reilly D, Oermann M. *Clinical Teaching in Nursing Education.* 2nd ed. NLN publication # 15-2471. New York: National League for Nursing; 1992.

Rogers C. *On Becoming a Person.* Boston: Houghton Mifflin; 1961.

Rogers ME. *The Theoretical Basis of Nursing.* Philadelphia: Davis; 1970.

Rosenstock IM. Why people use health services. *Milbank Memorial Fund.* 1966; 44:94–127.

Roy C, Roberts SL. *Theory Construction in Nursing: An Adaptation.* Englewood Cliffs, NJ: Prentice Hall; 1981.

Roy C, Andrews H. *The Roy Adaptation Model: The Definitive Statement.* Norwalk, CT: Appleton & Lange; 1991.

Selye H. *The Stress of Life.* New York: McGraw-Hill; 1956.

Smuts J. *Holism and Evolution.* New York: Macmillan; 1926.

Watson J. Postmodernism and knowledge development in nursing. *Nurs Sci Q.* 1995; 8:60–64.

World Health Organization. *Chronicle of the World Health Organization.* Geneva, Switzerland: WHO, Interim Commission; 1974.

BIBLIOGRAPHY

Erikson E. Eight stages of man. In: Lavatefli CS, Stendler F, eds. *Readings in Child Behavior and Child Development.* New York: Harcourt Brace Jovanovich; 1972.

Fowler J. Stages in Faith. In: Hennessy T, ed. *Values and Moral Development.* New York: Paulist Press; 1976.

Hadley BJ. Current concepts of wellness and illness: Their relevance for nursing. *Image.* 1974; 6:21–27.

Hamilton JM. Nursing and DRGs: Proactive responses to prospective reimbursement. *Nurs Health Care.* 1984; 5:155–160.

Havighurst RJ. *Human Development.* 2nd ed. New York: David McKay; 1972.

Huch M. Nursing in the next millennium. *Nurs Sci Q.* 1995; 8(1):38–44.

Kohlberg L. The development of moral thought. *Vita Humana.* 1963; 6:11.

Loevinger J. *Ego-Development: Conceptions and Theories.* San Francisco: Jossey-Bass; 1967.

Moccia P. *New Approaches to Theory Development* (New York: National League for Nursing; NLN publication #15–1992).

Patrick DC. Toward an operational definition of health. *J Health Soc Behav.* 1973; 14:62–63.

Quinn N, Somers A. The patient's bill of rights: A significant aspect of the consumer revolution. *Nurs Outlook*. 1974; 22:240.

Reed P. Framework for nursing knowledge development for the 21st century: Beyond postmodernism. *Adv Nurs Sci*. 1995; 17(3):70–84.

Rogers ME. The science of unitary man. In: Riehl JP, Roy C, eds. *Conceptual, Models for Nursing Practice*. 2nd ed. New York: Appleton-Century-Crofts; 1980.

Rosenstock IM. Historical origins of the health belief model. In: Becker MH, ed. *The Health Belief Model and Personal Health Behavior*. Thorofare, NJ: Slack; 1974.

Roy C. Developing nursing knowledge: Practice issues raised from four philosophical perspectives. *Nurs Sci Q*. 1995; 8(2):79–86.

Shaffer F. DRGs: History and overview. *Nurs Health Care*. 1983; 4:388–396.

White J. Patterns of knowing: Review, critique, and update. *Adv Nurs Sci*. 1995; 17(4):73–86.

Vincent P. The sick role in patient care. *Am J Nurs*. 1975; 75:1172.

2 CHAPTER

Major Theoretical Approaches to Nursing

▶ **Objectives**

After studying this chapter, the student will be able to:

1. List some theoretical foundations of the discipline of nursing.
2. State his or her own beliefs about central concepts of person, health, and environment.
3. List several definitions of nursing.
4. Describe some of the theoretical influences on nursing.
5. State four nurse theorists and their ideas of nursing's major concepts.

▶ **Questions to think about before reading the chapter**

- What are your personal beliefs and philosophy about nursing?
- What are some theories that influence nursing?
- What factors define nursing?
- Who are some nurse authors or theorists familiar to you?

▶ **Terms to know**

Developmental theory	Johnson, Dorothy
Entrophy	King, Imogene
Existentialism	Leininger, Madeline
Feedback	Needs theory
Henderson, Virginia	Negentrophy
Homeostasis	Neuman, Betty
Interpersonal process	Nightingale, Florence
Interpersonal theory	Orem, Dorothea

Orlando, Ida	Suprasystem
Peplau, Hildegarde	Systems theory
Phenomenology	Transition theory
Rogers, Martha	von Bertalanffy, Ludwig
Roy, Sister Callista	Wiedenbach, Ernestine
Subsystem	

▶ *Introduction*

Several theories and philosophies that have influenced nurse writers in their development of nursing theories are introduced in this chapter. Selected nurse theorists are then presented with their unique perspectives of nursing as well as their ideas of the concepts of person, health, and environment.

INFLUENCING THEORIES FOR NURSING THEORY DEVELOPMENT

Theories are developed as a result of many different thought processes and approaches. Most of the theoretical development in nursing has evolved from theories or paradigms outside the realm of nursing. Examples of these prototype theories or paradigms are systems theory, developmental theory, needs theory, interpersonal theory, phenomenology, and existentialist philosophy. Nurse theorists use varied approaches to develop and conceptualize their theories based on their unique views of the influencing theories, their individual views of concepts essential to nursing, and their personal experiences and ways of viewing the world.

It is important to realize that while the nurse theorists were influenced by other ideas, they reorganized and added new ideas to these paradigms in order to develop unique nursing perspectives, conceptual models, and theories. It was not enough for nurse theorists to simply borrow these theories from other fields and use them in nursing, since theories are developed for specific focuses of various fields and to adopt them unchanged into nursing's field would not be valid. Some of the influencing views for nursing theory development are addressed to illustrate backgrounds of the selected nurse theorists.

SYSTEMS THEORY

Systems theory is one method of conceptualizing the relationship of individuals, their environment, and health. Today many persons view systems theory and its related concepts as inherent to both the individual and groups of individuals. Systems concepts are derived from general systems theory as discussed by **Ludwig von Bertalanffy** (1968).

Systems

Systems theory offers an approach to the study of the person and the environment through the integration of various seemingly unconnected parts. It is a broad and all-encompassing approach, involving the interaction of the person and the environment as a whole. An underlying principle in this approach is that the whole is greater than and different from the sum of its parts. This means that, as various components interact, a unique blend is formed. The components by themselves would never have these properties. To make this definition more meaningful, consider these practical examples: you are more than the total of your physical makeup, and your family is more than the total of its members. Something additional occurs when your physical, psychological, cultural, and spiritual parts interact as a whole that makes you a unique person. The same is true of your family. With the interaction of the family members, a unique experience occurs that is different from the interaction of each of the members individually.

A system can also be an identified unit such as a client, group, society, or community. In viewing a system, it is essential that the component parts within the system (the **subsystem**) and those components outside the system (the **suprasystem**) be identified. Examples of the subsystem of a client are factors such as physical, psychological, sociological, cultural, and spiritual aspects, including values, beliefs, and aspirations. Suprasystems may include outside influences such as significant family members and friends, place and type of employment, health care facilities, and church and educational facilities. The interrelationship of the components of systems theory is depicted in Figure 2–1.

The broken lines in the diagram signify the open exchange of the system. Living systems may be considered relatively open in that they exchange energy–matter–information with the environment. Since this interaction is dynamic, any change in one part of the system will affect the entire system. The exchange of energy provides feedback to the system. In this manner, learning and change

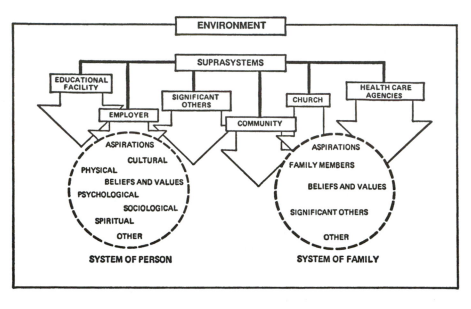

Figure 2–1. Structure of systems.

occur to maintain a dynamic balance, **homeostasis** or steady state, within and among the system, its subsystems, and suprasystems. Closed systems, unlike open systems, do not interact with the environment; therefore, all living systems are open.

The system continually receives input from the environment, reacts to it (throughout), produces output, and makes evaluations to adjust the input back into the system. This produces a process of feedback, diagrammed in Figure 2–2.

Systems, then, have identifiable structures. They also have a process—that is, systems interact with one another within boundaries that sort the input and output of the system. Input is information acquired by the system, throughput is information processing within the system, and output is information dispensed by the system. **Feedback** is a process of regulation for the system by which information concerning output is provided to the system. The state of organization within the system is referred to as **negentropy,** while the state of disorganization is referred to as **entropy.**

Developmental Theory

Developmental theorists have attempted to describe human development in terms of stages or changes that occur as individuals grow. The way these changes occur differs among the paradigms or views of the theorist. Some theorists believe change in the individual oc-

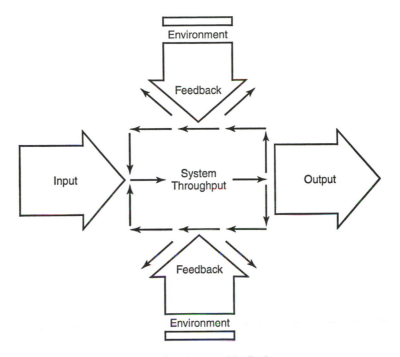

Figure 2–2. Process of feedback.

curs in smooth transitions, while others view change in stages and levels. The aspects of development viewed also vary among developmentalists. There is no one theory that encompasses all areas of human development. Some examples of **developmental theories** that have been used by nurse theorists in their development of theory are Piaget's theory of cognitive development; Erik Erikson's stages of psychosocial development; R. Havighurst's developmental tasks; James Fowler's stages of faith development; Kohlberg's stages of moral development; Loevinger's stages of ego development; and Levinson's stages of adult development. At every level of development, there are important tasks that must be mastered before progression can be made to the next developmental level. Other paradigms or views of development involve the importance and interaction of heredity and environment on personality.

Needs Theory

Many theorists have studied and described human **needs** that appear to be common to motivation and strivings of individuals. These motives or strivings direct behavior toward goal achievement. As with developmental theory, human needs theorists have varied in their view of important driving needs. Needs have been described in terms of biological needs and psychological needs. Some examples of biological needs are safety and pain; and stimulation and activity. Examples of psychological needs are order and predictability; adequacy and competence; love and affiliation; and values, meaning, and hope. Striving for actualization or fulfillment is another human need described by theorists. One of the best-known theorists in terms of needs and actualization is Maslow. He states that human needs are in a hierarchy where needs at the lowest level must be met before an individual can attend to higher level needs (see Chap. 1).

Interpersonal Theory

Interpersonal theory focuses on the individual as a social being. Harry Sullivan was one of the foremost theorists in this area. Sullivan believed that it is pointless to talk of individual personality since it does not exist apart from interaction with others.

Interpersonal process is the interaction between two or more people and is a key concept of interpersonal theory. The interpersonal process may be viewed from a number of conceptual approaches including a communication perspective. Many nurse theorists have focused on communication and interpersonal relationships in the development of their specific views of nursing.

In communication, a message is sent from one person or group to another, using some common set of symbols. The perception of the message is influenced by the experiences, knowledge, and sociocultural background of the receiver and the sender and the context in which the message is sent. Communication elicits feedback from the receiver. This process is illustrated in Figure 2–3. Nursing focuses on therapeutic communications or that which is goal-directed, purposeful, and contributes to a client's participation in progress toward a more healthy state.

For the process to be effective in nursing, nurses must have a personal awareness of their own beliefs, values, attitudes, and patterns of communication. One's beliefs, values, and attitudes have been shaped from one's experiences and influence one's perception of reality, behaviors, and interactions with others. Clients also have beliefs, values, and patterns of communication that they bring to the nurse–client interaction. Nurse–client values and beliefs interact in their impact on the communication process. Lack of awareness of one's own values or those of the client may result in communication blocks, which may lead to ineffective assessment and meeting of the client's needs.

The nurse–client interaction must be client-centered, involve the use of therapeutic communication skills, and must include client

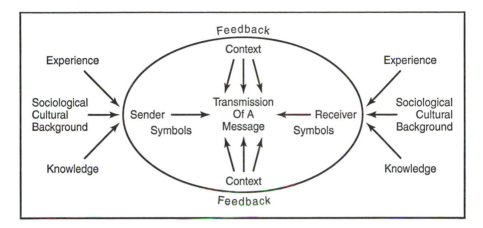

Figure 2–3. Communication process.

validation. Examples of therapeutic skills or techniques include focusing, facilitating, use of silence, use of therapeutic touch, and confrontation. Determination of the appropriate skills to use in a situation is based on data gathered from the assessment process as well as one's own skills and knowledge in communication. The interpersonal process looks at verbal and nonverbal behavior as a means of focusing on client feelings and concerns to determine client need and meet these needs more effectively. Although communication is used in all interactions, in the nurse–client relationship it is guided by therapeutic purposes and techniques.

Nursing involves the use of the interpersonal communication skills with clients to establish and meet health needs. It is essential that nurses look at the total person (physical, psychological, social, cultural, and spiritual) when establishing client needs. It is only through the integration of these aspects and recognition of the uniqueness of each individual that nurses can assist individuals toward optimum health levels.

Transition Theory

Transition is a concept that is currently investigated and talked about in nursing. Selder (1989) describes the **theory of life transition** as a process that bridges the disruption of reality to a newly constructed reality. It maintains the integrity of the person and sense of self. Meleis and Trangenstein (1994) identify transition as a central concept in nursing. They see transitions being related to or integral with such nursing concepts as Roy's adaptation, Orem's self-care, Roger's unitary human development, and Parse's expanding consciousness and human becoming. Chick & Meleis (1986) and Schumacher & Meleis (1994) define transition as a passage from one life phase or condition or status to another, a process and outcome of person–environment interactions. The three concur with the organizational theory that completion of transitions results in a period of greater stability and growth.

One example of a life transition is the period of life when a teenager becomes an adult. It is a transitional period of questioning one's life goals and of self-discovery. This disruptive period could begin with the completion of high school or the beginning of higher education and end with graduation and a sense of accomplishment. The transitional periods in an individual's life that are of interest to nursing *are those related to well-being* such as transition from health to unhealth within the family, transitions to parenthood, transitions to wellness, self concept transitions, changes in physical, emotional, or mental abilities. Nurses look for means to prevent unhealthy transitions.

Transitions usually encompass change but extend that concept to include the ideas of movement and flow. As Meleis explains it, the concept of change usually involves external changes, whereas transitions involve internal processes occurring over time.

Phenomenology

Phenomenology is a method of inquiry developed by Husserl (an early 1900s German philosopher), which involves an inspection of one's own conscious and intellectual processes. Merleau-Ponty was a French philosopher and phenomenologist (1908 to 1961) who investigated the relationship between consciousness and the world and rejected dualism of body and spirit. A phenomenon is a concept, idea, or event that is perceived by the senses. Phenomenalism analyzes physical object proposition and reduces all talk of things perceived to actual or possible perceived experiences. Both phenomenology and existentialism are philosophical views that have been the world view or basis of nurse theories.

Existentialism

Existentialism emphasizes the uniqueness of individuals, values and meaning, and self-direction and self-fulfillment of individuals. European philosophers such as Heidegger, Jaspers, Kierkegaard, and Sartre are especially influential to the development of this model. Existentials view the world as potentially dangerous, in which the individual's challenge is to establish personal identity and self-awareness in terms of his own experience and situation. Every individual must take the responsibility of making choices. The choosing of satisfying values is primary to individual essence. Individuals are inescapably the builders of personal life and existence by the freedom of choice, valuing, and personal accountability and responsibility.

Nurse Theorists

Nursing as a discipline must establish unique and common goals to give direction for the development of a body of knowledge. The uniqueness of the discipline of nursing is not in the sources of bodies of knowledge used but in the selection of the concepts from these sources in relation to the specific goals of the discipline.

Nurse theorists have organized their personal views of nursing's concepts of person, health, and environment into unique perspectives of the discipline having been influenced by views from many varied paradigms. Major concepts identified by nurse authors are shown in Tables 2–1 and 2–2.

TABLE 2–1. MAJOR CONCEPTS IDENTIFIED BY NURSING AUTHORS

Name	Concepts
Florence Nightingale, mid-1800s	Environmental conditions, health, and psychosocial factors
Hildegard Peplau, 1952	Interpersonal process; four major life tasks, psychodynamic nursing
Ernestine Wiedenbach, 1960	Three principles of helping; inconsistency–consistency, purposeful–perseverance, and self-extension; rational, reactionary, or deliberate nursing actions.
Virginia Henderson, 1960s	14 components of nursing care; independence; functioning
Dorothy Johnson, 1960–1980s	Behavioral system; external behavior force attachment–affiliative, dependency behavior, ingestion, elimination, sexuality, aggression, achievement
Ida Orlando, 1961	Patient, need, validation, interaction, health, improvement, nursing
Madeline Leininger, 1970s–1990s	Transcultural care model; caring, culture, cultural care, cultural care diversity, cultural care, universality care, social structure, health systems, cultural care maintenance, cultural care accommodation, cultural care repatterning
Betty Neuman, 1970s–1990s	Health care systems model; lines of defense, levels of prevention, stressors, individual variables, basic structure, reconstitution
Dorothea Orem, 1970–1990s	Self-care, conditioning factors, self-care agencies, self-care deficit, self-care demand, nursing systems
Imogene King, 1968–1990s	Personal, interpersonal, and social systems
Sr. Callista Roy, 1970s–1990s	Person as adaptive system, environment, health and goal of nursing
Martha Rogers, 1970–1990s	Principles of homeodynamics include resonancy, helicy, and integrality. Energy fields, negentropy, pattern, and four-dimensionality are other concepts.

Among the earliest individuals to organize nursing concepts was **Florence Nightingale.** Being a wealthy, educated woman, she was in a unique position in the mid-19th century to effect societal change. Though she did not use the terms "concept" or "theory," she expressed organized beliefs about nursing (Nightingale, 1940). Nightingale's unique education and experiences in a war-torn country were major influences in her organization of nursing knowledge. She was concerned with environmental conditions and individuals' physical, psychological, and social aspects and their relation to the health of the patient. Of prime importance was her view of nursing as a distinct discipline, separate from medicine.

Florence Nightingale in her book, *Notes on Nursing* (Nightingale, 1949, p. 133), described nursing as a process to put "the patient in the best condition for nature to act upon him." The environment must be conducive to health, with items such as hot water, fresh air, and cleanliness as means of putting the patient in the best condition. Florence Nightingale's contributions to nursing, which continue to have a major impact in nursing, are explored in more depth in Chapter 3.

Hildegard Peplau, writing in the 1950s, published what might be called a partial theory of nursing. Her theory focused primarily on her concept of the interpersonal process and the importance of purposeful patient–nurse interaction in the therapeutic healing process. According to Peplau, "Nursing is a significant, therapeutic, interpersonal process. It functions cooperatively with other human processes that make health possible for individuals in communities" (Peplau, 1952, p. 16). Peplau's original concept of the interpersonal process in nursing has four phases: orientation, identification, exploitation, and resolution. Her concepts concentrate on one aspect of nursing practice, the *interpersonal process.*

Ida Orlando developed a nursing model in 1961 in response to inadequate nursing care. Her model was one of the first to advocate validation of patient needs and patient participation in care. Orlando states the purpose of nursing is to supply help for a patient to have needs met. She identifies direct and indirect means of nursing activities. Orlando describes the basic core of nursing practice as understanding the interpersonal relationship between the nurse and the patient.

Ida Orlando, who wrote at a time when emphasis was placed on the interpersonal process, described nursing as helping to meet patient needs through the development of nurse–patient relationships. This definition, while contributing to one aspect of nursing, is limiting, since it focuses on a specific function of the nurse.

Ernestine Wiedenbach (1964) presented nursing as a clinical art that focuses on caring. Her theory is composed of three factors: central purpose, prescription, and realities. The central purpose is based on the nurse's philosophy. It defines the quality of care to be attained in the patient. Once a purpose is identified, the nurse works with the patient to develop a plan of care or prescription. Wiedenbach provides guidelines for viewing the realities of the situation in which nursing care is implemented.

Meleis (1991) speculates on developmental and phenomenological origins to this theory.

Another writer, **Virginia Henderson,** formulated nursing concepts in response to the many questions focusing around the basis or nature of nursing. The major questions of this time relate to the nurse practice acts, which are legal guidelines for the nurse's function in patient care. Prior to the period of Henderson's writing, a definition of nursing was essential to the formulation of nurse practice acts in legal terms. Henderson's concepts and theory of nursing were derived from her definition of nursing, (Henderson, 1966, p. 15).

Henderson identified 14 components that constitute basic nursing care. These components are assisting the individual with breathing normally; eating and drinking adequately; eliminating body waste; moving and maintaining desirable postures; sleeping and resting; selecting suitable clothes; maintaining body temperature; keeping the body clean, well-groomed, and protected; avoiding dangers in the environment; communicating with others in expressing emotions, needs, fears or opinions; worshipping according to one's faith; working with a sense of accomplishment; participating in various forms of recreation; learning, discovering, or satisfying the curiosity that leads to normal development and health; and using available health facilities.

Henderson believed that the nurse should be able to make independent judgments as long as medical diagnoses are not made, treatment for disease is not prescribed, or prognoses are not given. (The label of nursing diagnosis had not been formulated.) Her approach focuses on the individual person and human needs rather than solely on the environmental factors outlined by Nightingale. She focused on care of both ill and well individuals, using nursing practice to assist the person with independence.

Betty Neuman's systems model (1995) describes the interpersonal relationship between nurse and patient and the patient's response to stressors. Neuman uses a systems approach to guide the direction of professional health care. Her model is not intended for nurses only, but is for use by any health care professional. Neuman's model focuses on prevention of disease and the reaction of the patient to stressors or potential stressors in the environment. Neuman conceptualized the model as a systems approach to health care.

Madeline Leininger (1978) presents a unique perspective of nursing. Her model was developed from an anthropological technique. Dr. Leininger describes the component of care from the viewpoint of different cultures in order to delineate the essential components of care. This transcultural view is unique in nursing theory and nursing knowledge development. The essence of nursing, according to Dr. Leininger, is care. Care refers to "the assistive, supportive, or facilitative acts toward or for another individual or group with evident or anticipated needs, to ameliorate or improve the human condition or lifeway" (Leininger, 1984, p. 86). Leininger's sunrise model of transcultural diversity and university of care and health identifies three types of ethnonursing care: (1) care accommodations, (2) care preservation, and (3) care repatterning. Nursing care is a learned and scientific mode of enabling individuals and groups to provide culturally specific care to improve or maintain a health condition for life or death.

Dorothy Johnson developed a behavioral system model. She believes that nursing is a professional discipline and focuses on concepts of nursing and the person. The person is a behavior system comprising seven subsystems: attachment–affiliative, dependency, ingestive, eliminative, sexual, aggressive, and achievement. These behavior systems maintain their own integrity and link the individuals with the environment. Nursing problems are manifested when the subsystems cannot maintain the balance. Nursing is defined as the external regulating force that assists the individual to achieve system balance (Johnson, 1980).

Dorothea Orem (1991) is another nurse who has contributed to the body of nursing knowledge. Nursing is viewed as a means to assist individuals in the maintenance of self-care practices at various levels of health. She identifies three basic types of nursing systems: wholly compensatory, partly compensatory, and supportive-educative. There are varying nurse–patient (nurse–client) roles associated with each of the systems, and these roles are based on assessment of patient or client needs. In a wholly compensatory system, the nurse accomplishes the patient's (Orem's term) care. In this system, the nurse would give insulin injections to a patient newly diagnosed as having diabetes. As a patient progresses in the ability to administer injections, the nurse and patient move to a partly compensatory system. The patient would prepare the insulin and the nurse administer it in this system. In a supportive–educative system, the patient with diabetes would learn to give his or her own insulin injections following the nurse's instructions. This indicates that the patient accomplishes self-care, with the nurse and patient working together to overcome limitations.

The focus on individuals as active participants in their care is very similar to Henderson's views. Orem describes nursing as facilitating individuals' need for self-care, that is, activities that are initiated by persons with the goal of maintaining life, health, and well-being.

Toward a Theory in Nursing described the conceptualizations and definitions of nursing of **Imogene King** (1971, 1981). King focuses on persons as functioning within a social system through interpersonal relationships. Persons use their interpersonal relationships, which are influenced by perceptions, to maintain and define health. King (1971, p. 25) states that "nursing is a process of action, reaction, interaction and transaction whereby nurses assist individuals of any age and socioeconomic group to meet their basic needs in performing activities of daily living and to cope with health and illness at some particular point in the life cycle."

Sister Callista Roy also uses a systems approach and views the person as a biopsychosocial being continually adapting to the environment. Four adaptive modes are identified: (1) physiological needs, (2) self-concept, (3) role function, and (4) interdependency. The nursing role is to assess the client's behavior and to assist the individual to adapt successfully to change (Roy, 1976, 1991).

The final author to be considered is **Martha Rogers** (1970), who focused on nursing as a science. She perceived the person as central to nursing's purpose. Her theoretical focus was on "a science of unitary man." Using a systems perspective, she described nursing as a humanistic science that can explain and predict the nature and development of individuals. Rogers identified nursing as both a science and an art. The purpose of nursing is to help people achieve maximum well-being within the potential of the self and group. Nursing involves an integrality of continuous diversity patterning of human fields.

Martha Rogers viewed the person as a unified whole coexisting with the environment. Rogers drew from the knowledge of many disciplines, including anthropology, sociology, religion, philosophy, history, and astronomy. Her approach was both futuristic and holistic. Rogers described nursing as a science whose purpose is to describe and explain the life processes of humankind. These are processes that are inseparable from the environment. She described health and illness as "expressions of the process of life" (p. 85). Rogers stated that nursing aims to "provide a body of abstract knowledge ... capable of being translated into nursing practice" (p. 86). Rogers identified the unique individual way of practice as the art of nursing that draws from the scientific principles basic to the discipline. She viewed noninvasive modalities as characteristic

TABLE 2–2. SUMMARY OF DEFINITIONS OF PERSON, ENVIRONMENT, AND HEALTH BY NURSE THEORISTS

Name	Person	Environment	Health
Florence Nightingale	Physical, intellectual, and spiritual being	Physical elements that affect the healing process	Addictive process, result of psychological, physical, and environmental factors
Hildegard Peplau	Individual with potential for growth	External factors and significant others	Linked to development; forward movement of personality and human processes
Ernestine Wiedenbach	Functioning being; presented using four basic assumptions concerning human nature	Not explicated in this model	Not explicated in this model
Virginia Henderson	Biological being, oneness of mind and body	Not explicated in this model	Ability to function independently
Dorothy Johnson	Biological, abstract system with seven behavioral-centered needs and tasks	All factors not directly part of the individual behavior system	Balance, state of stability and moving state of equilibrium, elusive state comprised of psychological, social, and physiological factors
Dorothea Orem	Self-care entity that seeks to maintain or promote optimal health. Unique in ability to reflect and symbolize.	Includes psychosocial and physical entities, as well as attitudes, abilities, and self-concept	State of wholeness or integrity
Imogene King	Open systems who are rational, sentient, time-oriented, social beings, exhibiting common characteristics and interacting	Internal and external elements involving temporal and spatial reality	Dynamic life experiences involving continuous adjustment to stressors to achieve maximum potential for daily living

Theorist	Person	Environment	Health
Betty Neuman	Open system composed of physiological, psychological, sociocultural, and developmental variables	Both internal and external	Equilibrium steady-normal line of defense
Sr. Callista Roy	Open, adaptive system involving input, internal processes (regulator and cognator), feedback, and output. Adaptive goals of the person are survival, growth, reproduction, and mastery in regard to the four modes.	Conditions, circumstances, and influence that surround and affect the person (focal conceptual residual stimuli)	A state and process of being and becoming "an integrated and whole person"
Martha Rogers	Unified whole possessing integrity and manifesting characteristics that are more than and different from the sum of the parts. Open system in constant interaction with the environment	Patterned wholeness of all that is human. An irreducible, four-dimensional energy field	Health is described as ease versus disease. A continuum that is arbitrarily defined, culturally infused, and value laden
Ida Orlando	Behaving human organism	Nursing setting	Mental and physical comfort adequacy or well-being
Madeline Leininger	Cultural beings	Social structure	State of well-being that enables one to perform activities or achieve life goals

of the next phase within nursing. She stated that the Krieger-Kunz method of therapeutic touch and humor are examples of noninvasive therapy that is currently being used to great advantage in nursing. With the change to community-based health care, well-being should be the focus and unique phenomenon of nursing.

Each of these nursing writers has contributed to the expanding body of nursing knowledge and practice that constitutes the discipline of nursing. However, as yet, none of the authors has met all the criteria of theory development. The challenge to nursing, therefore, remains to develop these concepts into theories that will continue to promote nursing as a discipline. It is important to realize that nurses are making contributions to theory development. Only a few of these nurses have been presented in this section of the chapter. Table 2–3 offers a summary of current definitions of nursing.

TABLE 2–3. SUMMARY OF CURRENT DEFINITIONS OF NURSING

Name	Nursing
Florence Nightingale, mid 1800s	A calling; discover and use nature's laws regarding health.
Hildegard Peplau, 1952	Significant, therapeutic interpersonal process.
Ernestine Wiedenbach, 1960	Four elements of clinical nursing, philosophy (way), purpose (why), practice (what), and art (how).
Ida Orlando, 1961	Helping to meet patient needs through nurse–patient relationships.
Virginia Henderson, 1960s	Assisting individuals in performance of those activities contributing to health or its recovery; defined in terms of 14 components of nursing care; practice-centered.
Dorothy Johnson, 1960–1980s	External regulatory force to organize and integrate client behavior and assist in maintaining balance.
Dorothea Orem, 1969–1990s	Helping service that assists individuals toward designing, providing, and managing systems of therapeutic self-care.
Imogene King, 1968–1990s	Process of action, reaction, and interaction where nurse and clients share information to assist clients to maintain health and function in their roles.
Sr. Callista Roy, 1970s–1990s	Goal is to promote adaptation in regard to the four adaptive modes (physical, self-concept, role function, and interdependence).
Martha Rogers, 1970–1990s	Exists to serve people. Committed to maintaining and providing evaluative, therapeutic, and rehabilitative services.
American Nurses Association, 1980	Diagnosis and treatment of human responses to actual or potential health problems.
Betty Neuman, 1970s–1990s	Reduction of stress factors to affect optimal functioning through primary, secondary, and tertiary prevention.
Madeline Leininger, 1970–1990s	Culturally based profession involving professional caring actions made to assist, support, or facilitate another person or group with a need to improve or ameliorate a human condition or lifeway.

As we have seen, throughout nursing's history, nursing leaders have attempted to delineate factors that describe nursing. Nurse theorists have responded to the need to define nursing in terms other than activities, or tasks that the nurse accomplishes. They have defined nursing in the context of their individual paradigm or theory and have focused on the content and process of nursing rather than personal characteristics of the nurse.

SUMMARY

Nursing discipline is based on unique perspectives of person, health, and environment as identified by theories unique to nursing and theories outside nursing. Throughout the history of nursing, the identification of the unique perspective of nursing has been a challenge to nurse scholars. This chapter has introduced theories used by nurse scholars to conceptualize the uniqueness and essence of nursing. Several nurse authors have been identified and an overview provided of their conceptualization of the focus of nursing.

▶ Questions for Discussion

1. What contributions have nurse theorists made to the discipline of nursing?
2. Why is it important to look at theory in relation to nursing?
3. Which theorist's ideas are most like yours in terms of nursing?
4. How has your definition of nursing changed since reading this chapter?
5. How can systems theory be related to nursing?

REFERENCES

Chick N, Meleis AI. Transitions: A nursing concern. In: Chinn PL, ed. *Nursing Research Methodology: Issues and Implementation.* Rockville, MD: Aspen Systems; 1986:237–257.

Henderson V. *The Nature of Nursing.* New York: Macmillan; 1966.

Johnson DE. The behavioral system model for nursing. In: Riehl, JP, Roy, C, eds. *Conceptual Models for Nursing Practice.* New York: Appleton-Century-Crofts; 1980.

King, I. *A Theory for Nursing.* New York: Wiley; 1978.

King, I. *A Theory for Nursing: Systems, Concepts, Process.* New York: John Wiley; 1987.

Leininger M. *Transcultural Nursing Concepts, Theories, and Practices.* New York: Wiley; 1978.

Leininger M. *Care, the Essence of Nursing and Health.* Thorofare, NJ: Slack; 1984.

Meleis A. *Theoretical Nursing: Development and Process.* 2nd ed. Philadelphia: Lippincott; 1991.

Meleis A, Trangenstein P. Facilitating transitions: Redefinition of the nursing mission. *Nurs Outlook.* 1994; 42:255–259.

Merton R. On sociological theories of the middle range. In: *On theoretical sociology,* New York: The Free Press; 1977.

Neuman B. *The Neuman Systems Model.* 3rd ed. Norwalk, CT: Appleton & Lange; 1995.

Nightingale F. *Notes on Nursing.* New York: Appleton-Century-Crofts; 1940.

Orem D. *Nursing: Concepts of Practice.* 4th ed. St. Louis: Mosby Year Book; 1991.

Orlando I. *The Dynamic Nurse–Patient Relationship,* New York: Putnam; 1961.

Peplau H. *Interpersonal Relations in Nursing.* New York: Putnam; 1952.

Rogers ME. *The Theoretical Basis of Nursing.* Philadelphia: Davis; 1970.

Rogers M. The science of unitary human beings: Current perspectives. *Nurs Sci Q.* 1994; 7(1):33–5.

Roy C. *Introduction to Nursing: An Adaptation Model.* Englewood Cliffs, NJ: Prentice-Hall; 1976.

Roy C. *Introduction to Nursing: An Adaptation Model.* 2nd ed. Englewood Cliffs, NJ: Prentice-Hall; 1994.

Roy C, Andrews H. *The Roy Adaptation Model: The Definitive Statement.* Norwalk, CT: Appleton & Lange; 1991.

Selder F. Life transition theory: The resolution of uncertainty. *Nurs Health Care.* 1989; 10(8):437–451.

Schumacher KL, Meleis AI. 1994. Transitions: a central concept in nursing. *Image.* 1995; 26(2):119–127.

von Bertalanffy L. *General Systems Theory: Foundations, Development, and Application.* New York: George Braziller; 1968.

Widenbach E. *Clinical Nursing: A Helping, Art.* New York: Springer; 1964.

BIBLIOGRAPHY

Barrett E. *Visions of Roger's Science-Based Nursing.* New York: National League for Nursing; 1990:15–2285.

Benoliel J. The interaction between theory and research. *Nurs Outlook.* 1977; 25(21):108–113.

Bohny BJ. Theory development for a nursing science. *Nurs Forum.* 1980; 19(1):57–67.

Brooks JA, Kleine-Kracht A. Evolution of a definition of nursing. *Adv Nurs Sci* (1983); 6:51–63.

Bruner J. *Toward a Theory of Instructions.* Cambridge, MA: Belknap Press; 1966.

Chinn P, Kramer M. *Theory and Nursing: A Systematic Approach.* 3rd ed. St. Louis: Mosby Year Book; 1991.

Conway M. Toward greater specificity in defining nursing's metaparadigm. *Adv Nurs Sci.* 1985; 7(4):73–81.

Daubenmire M, King I. Nursing process models: A systems approach. *Nurs Outlook.* 1971; 21:512–517.

Dennis K, Prescott P. Florence Nightingale: Yesterday, today, and tomorrow. *Adv Nurs Sci.* 1985; 66:66–81.

Dickoff J, James P. A theory of theories: A position paper. *Nurs Res.* 1968; 17:197–201.

Dickoff J, Wiedenbach E. Theory in a practice discipline. *Nurs Res.* 1968; 17:415–435.

Ellis R. Characteristics of significant theories. *Nurs Res.* 1968; 17:217–222.

Engstrom J. Problems in the development, use and testing of nursing theory. *J Nurs Educ.* 1984; 23:245–251.

Erikson E. Eight stages of man. In: Lavatelli CS, Stendler F, eds. *Readings in Child Behavior and Child Development.* New York: Harcourt Brace Jovanovich; 1972.

Fawcett J. Hallmarks of success in nursing theory development. In: Chinn P, ed. *Advances in Nursing Theory Development.* Rockville, MD: Aspen Systems; 1983.

Fawcett J. *Analysis and Evaluation of Conceptual Models of Nursing.* Philadelphia: Davis; 1984.

Fitzpatrick J, Whall A. *Conceptual Models of Nursing Analysis and Application.* 2nd ed. Norwalk, CT: Appleton & Lange; 1989.

Flaskerud J, Halloran E. Areas of agreement in nursing theory development. *Adv Nurs Sci.* (1980); 3:1–7.

Fowler J. Stages in faith: The structural-developmental approach. In: Hennessy T, ed. *Values and Moral Development.* New York: Paulist Press; 1976.

Fulton J. Virginia Henderson: Theorist, prophet, poet. *Adv Nurs Sci.* 1987; 10:1–9.

Hardy ME. Perspectives on nursing theory. *Adv Nurs Sci.* 1978; 1:37–48.

Johnson D. The nature of a science of nursing. *Am J Nurs.* 1959; 59:291–294.

Johnson D. Development of theory: A requisite for nursing as a primary health profession. *Nurs Res.* 1974; 18:372–377.

Kuhn TS. *The Nature of Scientific Revolution.* 2nd ed. Chicago: University of Chicago Press; 1970.

Lancaster W, Lancaster J. Models and model building in nursing. *Adv Nurs Sci.* 1981; 3:31–42.

Lazarus RS. *Psychological Stress and the Coping Process.* New York: McGraw-Hill; 1966.

Newman MA. The continuing revolution: A history of nursing science. In: Chasta N, ed. *The Nursing Profession: A Time to Speak.* New York: McGraw-Hill; 1983: 385–393.

Orlando I. *The Dynamic Nurse-Patient Relationship.* New York: Putnam; 1962.

O'Toole AW, Welt SR. *Interpersonal Theory in Nursing Practice: Selected Works of Hildegard E. Peplau.* New York: Springer; 1989.

Rawnsley M. Health, a Rogerian perspective. *J Holistic Nurs.* 1983; 3:1.

Rogers M. *An Introduction to the Theoretical Basis of Nursing.* Philadelphia: Davis; 1970.

Rogers ME. The science of unitary man. In: Riehl JP, Roy C, eds. *Conceptual Models for Nursing Practice.* 2nd ed. New York: Appleton-Century-Crofts; 1980.

Riehl-Sisca J. *Conceptual Models for Nursing Practice.* 3rd ed. Norwalk, CT: Appleton & Lange; 1989.

Selye H. *The Stress of Life.* New York: McGraw-Hill; 1956.

Silva MC, Rothhart D. An analysis of changing trends in philosophies of science on nursing theory and development testing. *Adv Nurs Sci.* 1984; 6:1–13.

Walker L, Avant K. *Strategies for Theory Development in Nursing.* 2nd ed. Norwalk, CT: Appleton & Lange; 1988.

Historical Development of the Discipline of Nursing and Nursing Education

▸ **Objectives**

After studying the chapter, the student will be able to:

1. Describe the historical development of nursing from pre-Christian to present times.
2. Trace the evolution of nursing programs in the United States.
3. Compare the three types of educational programs for basic preparation as a registered nurse.
4. Describe the implications of the various landmark studies on nursing and nursing education.
5. Discuss various themes evident in nursing history.

▸ **Questions to think about before reading the chapter**

- What do you know about Florence Nightingale?
- Can you name some past and present leaders in nursing?
- What are the ongoing educational trends for preparation for nursing practice?
- What impact have wars, increased technology, religion, women's movement, and the consumer movement had on nursing?

▸ **Terms to know**

American Association of Colleges of Nursing (AACN)

American Nurses Association (ANA)

ANA Position Paper

Associate degree

Baccalaureate degree

Brown Report (*Nursing for the Future*)

Community or junior college

Critical thinking

Diploma in nursing

Doctor's degree

Goldmark Report (*Nursing and Nursing Education in the United States*)

Graduate education

Lysaught Report (*Abstract for Action*)

Master's degree

Montag, Mildred

National Commission on Nursing

National League for Nursing (NLN)

Nightingale, Florence

PEW

Surgeon General's Report (*Toward Quality in Nursing*)

Wald, Lillian

▶ *Introduction*

To appreciate and understand modern nursing, it is necessary to have an idea of nursing's beginnings, its struggle for autonomy, and some of the leaders and events that have led to the development of the present-day discipline. Viewing nursing from a historical perspective can provide an understanding of issues and trends in nursing and provide a foundation to predict future events.

This chapter focuses on some of the issues and trends in nursing history that have influenced nursing history and nursing education. Since the pre-Christian era, various recurring forces have influenced nursing and health care. Some of these include religious and spiritual beliefs, the military and wars, changes in technology and scientific advances, social issues, the health care crisis, and the role of women and nursing.

THE PRE-CHRISTIAN ERA

Nursing as it is known today was first conceptualized by **Florence Nightingale** in the mid-1800s. Before that time, nursing was not clearly identified. There is evidence that in prehistoric times, someone provided nurturing, care, and comfort to the sick and injured (Fitzpatrick, 1983). The actual role of nursing in these early civilizations is not clear, but what is evident is the intermingling of nursing and medicine, both being referred to under the term "medicine." Treatments and healing were primarily the responsibility of village medicine men and practitioners of witchcraft. Religion has also been closely linked to medicine throughout civilization, with priests, priestesses, or shamans (witch doctors) in ancient times often the ones responsible for healing practices. Early civilizations thought spirits had a role in health. The supernatural was used to explain the development of a fever or sudden illness that was not readily attributed to the effects of an injury, such as a bruise from a fall. Magic and superstition surrounded the practice of medicine in these ancient cultures. Evil spirits were commonly thought to be the cause of illness, and many incantations, surgical practices, and potions were developed to drive them out and rid the body of disease. These beliefs gave rise to the role of the physician-shaman, who held a high position of authority.

Nursing evolved in response to the basic needs of life. Within each household, women were the creators of life and cared for their own. They were frequently summoned to care for others in the community who were ill. Often they were considered servants or slaves, occupying a very subservient and dependent role. Within their houses they were not free, and certainly not free to be educated. For the most part, women learned the art of healing and passed it to their daughters. Nursing was consistent with, not separate from, life.

As civilization developed, there were changes in society that affected medicine and nursing. One culture that made a significant contribution was the Egyptian. The Egyptian physicians such as Imhotep, who was honored as a god after his death, introduced the practice of embalming, classified 250 different diseases, and developed the drugs and treatments needed in the care of these diseases. In spite of the advances, magic and the beliefs in evil spirits so permeated early philosophies that there was little change in medicine or health care.

A new awakening in human thought and attitudes brought on by the Greeks led to changes in society that affected medicine and nursing. Hippocrates of Cos (ca. 460 to 370 B.C.), a Greek scholar, was the most advanced physician of his time. He changed medicine from superstitious magic into a science by stressing the use of the senses for assessment and gathering facts to make a diagnosis. He outlined plans of care for patients based on diseases being caused by the environment, not the gods. His writings were in a textbook of medicine that was used for many years. Hippocrates is often referred to as the "father of modern medicine" and many medical colleges today have their graduates take the Oath of Hippocrates as an ethical guide to medical conduct.

Greek medicine was divided into two groups: secular medicine, which was headed by Hippocrates; and the older religious medicine, which had the god of healing, Asklepios, as its leader. (Asklepios is the oldest spelling. Others include Asclepius or the Latin form, Aesculapius.) An emblem for medicine was developed, called a *caduceus,* which comes from Asklepios; the word means snakelike. This emblem depicts the staff of a traveler intertwined with a serpent (representing wisdom) and the wings from the feet of Mercury; the messenger of the gods. Asklepios had five children, two of whom were the first women to be associated with medicine: Hygeia, goddess of health, and Panacea, restorer of health. Very little was known about nursing during this time; however, there is evidence that Hippocrates wanted educated nurses to care for patients at the bedside, not the "slave nurse." The nurses of this time were probably either men or women who attended to the sick in the home or in health resorts of spas.

The ancient Hebrews contributed to health care with both their Mosaic health code, which included principles of hygiene, rest, nutrition, and other health-promoting behaviors such as Kosher preparation of foods to decrease the possible contamination that could occur by mixing meat and dairy products. The Ten Commandments provide guidelines for a code of ethics.

Another civilization important to medicine and nursing was that of the Romans. Rome's contributions were not to medicine, but to nursing through its use of nurses in the military (Bullough & Bullough, 1984). As a result of Rome's military conquests, medicine and nursing were carried to other areas of the Roman world, including the Mediterranean. As the Roman Empire collapsed, much of the health care knowledge that had been developed was lost.

During this pre-Christian period, nursing remained predominantly in homes, with care restricted to the sick. Contributions of women to health care were considered minimal, since the physician-shaman had become associated with authority and spiritual powers. Nurses assumed a subservient role, taking direction from physicians. Nursing moved away from the educational realm into the religious area, where there was little intellectual emphasis.

THE CHRISTIAN ERA

Religion, medicine, and nursing were again intertwined with the advent of Jesus Christ. Many nursing functions developed as groups of persons such as deaconesses, matrons, and widows visited and cared for the sick and needy in their homes in response to Christ's teaching of love and individual responsibility. Many hospitals were built as places to care for the sick and the poor, especially during epidemics.

During this era there were several significant women identified as contributors in the development of nursing. Phoebe was one of the best known of the Roman deaconesses of the early church and is often referred to as one of the first visiting nurses. St. Helena, Marcella, Fabiola, and Paula were other famous Roman matrons. Helena, the mother of Constantine the Great, gave abundantly to the sick and needy and helped to build hospitals for the elderly. Marcella established a monastery in her home where she taught the care of the sick and encouraged the intellectual development of women. Fabiola, a follower of Marcella, converted her place into the first Christian hospital in Rome and worked there in the care of the sick. Paula was an aristocrat and a very educated woman. She is recognized for her collegial relationship with scholarly men and for building shelters for the sick. As a result of the work of these wealthy, educated women, Christian hospitals were established throughout the Mediterranean lands.

During the 12th century, Hildegarde, another significant woman, contributed to the scientific foundation for nursing and medicine. She required her female students to wear a uniform and veil, which signified humility, obedience, and service. The veil was replaced by the nurse's cap. These esteemed women were of high social standing and probably were the forerunners of modern nurses.

Three formal organizations of nurses developed in the Middle Ages that influenced nursing today: the military, religious, and secular orders. During the Crusades (1096 to 1291) there was an increased need for hospitals and health care providers. To meet these needs, military nursing orders were developed. These orders attracted men who were carefully screened and then recognized as knights. These nurse-knights were used in battle as well as in the hospitals. One famous military order was The Knights Hospitallers of St. John of Jerusalem (Knights of Malta). Many religious orders developed in response to health care needs caused by the plagues as well as increased devotion to following the teachings of Christ. Some of the religious orders founded at this time were by Saints Francis of Assisi (Franciscans), Dominic (Dominicans), Clare (Poor Clares), and Catherine. The members of secular orders cared for the sick but did not take religious vows. Some of these lay persons were independent; others were organized under the auspices of the church. Both groups carried out works of charity that often included care of the sick. Much of nursing became secularized by the 14th century.

In the general education movement of this period, new philosophies formed, and stores of knowledge were developed. Hospitals continued to develop throughout the 15th century. Patients were cared for by educated male and female nurses. The era of the Renaissance (1438 to 1600) was a time of revival of learning. Universities began to appear in Europe. Medicine moved into the university setting, but nursing remained within religious and military orders.

The high level of nursing care that prevailed up to this time was lost during the Reformation (16th century). During the Reformation, religious orders were suppressed; churches, monasteries, and hospitals closed; nursing orders were disbanded; and virtually all males disappeared from nursing. Hospitals began to reopen as illness and the bubonic plague spread over Europe, but nursing had lost its social status and the nurses in the hospital were lower-class women, often poorly educated, or criminals serving sentences. Nursing was considered a last-resort occupation for women when they could no longer make a living from crime and prostitution. A woman's place was in the home, and no respectable woman would have a career. Thus, nursing was without organization, education, or social status. This was considered the darkest age for nursing, and it persisted until well into the 18th century.

Society's attitudes about nursing are reflected in the writings of Charles Dickens (1812 to 1870), a man keenly aware of societal needs. His book, *Martin Chuzzlewit* (1844) (Dickens, 1896), refers to the nursing care given by criminals and women of low moral standards. Sairey Gamp, the central figure in this book, was an alcoholic nurse often cited as the worst example of her profession. The portrayal greatly influenced attitudes toward nurses and nursing.

The Industrial Revolution, which began in England and France in the mid-18th century and in Germany and the United States in the 19th, also affected nursing. With the Industrial Revolution, the impact of machinery, the factory, and consequent developments contributed to undesirable working conditions and negative attitudes toward the working class. The negative societal effects of the Industrial Revolution were reflected in the health status of workers. Poor working conditions, poverty, long hours, and child labor were just a few of the negative effects of this period. In addition, there was indifference toward health care, and care methods and attitudes were inhumane. Several individuals and groups responded to the deplorable health conditions in an attempt to raise social consciousness and effect change. More hospitals were opened to care for the increase in people with illnesses and injuries from the working conditions. Caring for the sick became more socially acceptable as the middle class began to develop, blurring the distinction between the upper and lower class. Women began to be emancipated and take on roles that were once taboo for any respectable woman.

In reviewing the historical development of nursing, we see that the changing role of women has been a predominant factor. Indeed, perhaps the strongest single inhibiting factor for nursing arose out of societal attitudes toward women.

For many centuries, women remained in the home and cared for the children. They were not offered the opportunity for education. While women were in the home, men were actively involved in educational endeavors that eventually became localized in institutions of higher learning.

The image or self-concept of women was marked by sexism and subservience to male domination without autonomy. In most instances, this led to women's failure to assume leadership positions. Nursing developed out of health needs within the home, where women were situated. This led to the development of the caring aspect of nursing.

Although the caring element is essential to nursing, the profession lacked the knowledge and educational base at this period that would give nursing its unique theory and research position. During the late 18th and early 19th centuries, medical knowledge continued to expand, and women interested in social reform established lay organizations (e.g., the St. Vincent de Paul Society) and religious nursing institutions.

Before this, there were no schools for preparing nurses. In 1836, in response to growing social needs, Theodor Fliedner, a Lutheran pastor, and his wife, Frederike, started a center to train women as deaconesses at Kaiserwerth, Germany, to care for the sick. The pupils were from many countries, including England. The school included practical, theoretical, and code of conduct material. The students wore uniforms and were formally instructed in caring for both sick and convalescent adults and children, the administration of medications, and religious work. Students were carefully selected on the basis of references from clergymen and physicians. This Kaiserwerth training school model gave much inspiration to Florence Nightingale, and her schools incorporated many of the educational practices used at Kaiserwerth.

The establishment of a formal training school was a positive step for nursing. However, unlike that of physicians, the education of nurses remained outside the formal university setting. It remained for nurses to convince not only hospital administrators, physicians, and educators of the importance of nursing, but more crucially, to convince women themselves and the general public.

MODERN NURSING

Influence of Florence Nightingale

Until the 1800s, nursing had been closely connected with church-related organizations and hospitals. Nursing was not organized into a profession, and the training of nurses did not rest on educational principles, patient needs, or health-based practices. Most of the training was apprenticeship; nurses were taught techniques that had worked in the past rather than skills based on scientific knowledge or research findings. Florence Nightingale was to initiate change in this type of training and thus alter the whole structure and concept of what nursing is and what it should become.

As previously discussed, many people were feeling the need for social reform in the 1800s. Prisons and hospitals were in deplorable condition. It was at this time that the founder of modern nursing, Florence Nightingale (1820 to 1910) (Fig. 3–1) was born to a wealthy, educated English family. She was educated in philosophy, languages, and other liberal arts. During the mid-1800s, she visited many hospitals and studied various nursing systems. Although Nightingale was interested in helping and caring for others as a nurse, nursing still was not a respected profession at this time in history. After caring for family members during illness, she became more convinced of the need for education in nursing as well as the aspects of caring and concern traditionally associated with nursing. In 1851, at the age of 31, and after considerable family dissension, Nightingale obtained her parents' consent to enter nursing training at Kaiserwerth. She had practiced nursing in English hospitals up until this time.

She spent 3 months studying under the Fliedners at Kaiserwerth and then continued her studies with the Sisters of Charity of St. Vincent de Paul in Paris. After her studies, she became the superintendent of the Establishment for Gentlewomen During Illness. Her goal was to change the social view of nurses from the low-life "Sairey Gamp" type to that of well-educated caregivers.

With the persuasion of Dr. Bowman, a famous surgeon of the day, she became the superintendent of nurses in the King's College Hospital in England until she left for Scutari to assist with the wounded in the Crimean War (1854 to 1856). The casualties in this war were very high, and the care of the wounded was deplorable. The English felt a need for nurses to care for the wounded. Sidney Herbert, the secretary of war in 1854 and a personal friend of Nightingale, asked her to come to Crimea, where she assumed the role of Superintendent of the Female Nursing Establishment of the English General Hospitals in Turkey. During the war, she was able to prepare about 40 nurses to care for 1500 patients who were in war hospitals under wretched conditions. She reduced the mortality rate from almost 50 percent to just 2 percent by initiating care based on principles of cleanliness and nutrition. Nightingale also organized all the hospitals throughout Crimea and kept extensive records of her experiences.

It was during the Crimean War that Florence Nightingale became known as the "lady with the lamp." She made the rounds to the wounded soldiers at night with a lantern and became a source of comfort. Longfellow immortalized her in his poem "The Lady with

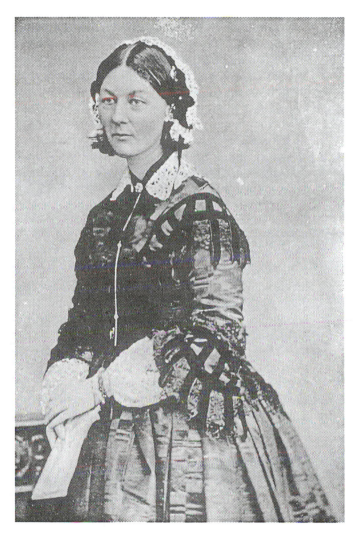

Figure 3–1. Florence Nightingale. *(Florence Nightingale Museum, London.)*

the Lamp." However, she did more than this. It was through her efforts that hospital conditions greatly improved in this outpost station. She used her own money and personal influence to get the supplies and the facilities needed for the improvement of health care. During this time, Nightingale became ill with the Crimean fever, which was probably typhoid or typhoid fever. This disease left her weak, and she never completely recovered from it.

In 1859, Florence Nightingale published a book entitled *Notes on Nursing: What It Is and What It Is Not*. The contents of her book came from data collected during her years of nursing and from her travels. Her book was widely distributed and translated into three languages. It contained guidelines for personal hygienic practices and her ideas of what nursing was all about. Nightingale stated "that to be well is the purpose of all being" (Nightingale, 1940, p. 45), and she recognized individual differences, believing in "scope for individual exercises of idiosyncrasy" (p. 46). She transcended the boundaries of hospital nursing, believing that the purpose of nursing was not only hospital care of the sick but helping people to live.

In 1860, the Nightingale Training School for Nurses became a reality as a result of a gift of money given to Nightingale by the British nation in gratitude for her contribution during the Crimean War. The school was opened at St. Thomas' Hospital in London. The opening of the school was not favored by London physicians, who saw nurses as maids who could cook and attend to cleanliness. Because of Nightingale's ill health, Sarah Wardroper, a stern and capable woman, was selected as the matron of the school. Admission requirements were highly selective, and only 15 students were admitted to the program from over 1000 applicants. Nightingale believed that nurses should be prepared in broad fields of liberal education prior to entering nursing. She believed nurses needed to be well-bred and formally educated to provide better care for the patients. Her curriculum consisted of anatomy, medicine, surgery, physiology, chemistry, and nutrition.

Nightingale developed principles of nursing education, which included (1) the training school should be an educational institution supported by public funds and associated with a medical school; (2) it should be affiliated with a teaching hospital but also independent of it; (3) professional nurses should be in charge of administration and instruction; and (4) there should be a home for the students in order to maintain discipline and character (Notter & Spalding, 1976). Nightingale believed that the school should be an educational and not a service institution for the hospital. This issue continued to be debated for many years after Nightingale's death.

Florence Nightingale made many suggestions for improving care of patients. She stressed the ideas of fresh air, medications, quiet, mobility, piped hot water, a call-bell system for patients, cleanliness, and comfort in the hospitals, as well as educating the public concerning health and illness. These improvements helped to upgrade nursing to a socially acceptable position. Nightingale directed the training of nurses, who were referred to as "the Nightingale nurses," in public health, public reform, and health promotional aspects of nursing and also the care of the sick.

With the belief that schools of nursing should be separate from hospitals, graduates of the Nightingale school were sent out to become matrons of other schools. After 1900, complex political, societal, and economical influences resulted in expansion of these schools into diploma programs under the auspices of the hospital rather than within institutions of higher education. These programs are referred to as hospital schools of nursing.

The evolution of nursing and nursing education are closely linked. Major themes of social influences are reflected in the development of nursing education. During the time of Florence Nightingale, medical schools, clinics, and community agencies were being developed throughout Europe.

Nursing in America

Until the 1800s, health care, medicine, and nursing followed European patterns. Early nursing care in America was delivered in the home. Hospitals became more prominent in the 17th and 18th centuries as places to treat contagious diseases (Kalisch & Kalisch, 1986). Medical knowledge was beginning to develop in the United States, although Philadelphia was the only city of medical renown during most of the 18th century. The first hospital was started there in 1751.

For the most part, institutions had developed structurally to be male dominated. Therefore, as women moved out of the home into institutions, they were moving into another position subservient to male administrators and boards of trustees.

In 1839, the first attempt at an organized school of nursing in America was started by the Nurse Society of Philadelphia under Dr. Joseph Warrington. The program trained women by the use of manikins, and Dr. Warrington's classes were taught together with medical students. These women were given a "certificate of approbation" at the end of their training (Jenson, et al., 1955).

During the mid-1800s the role of women was still in the home. They were uneducated and unable to pursue careers outside of the home. Men considered women mentally and physically inferior because of their smaller, more delicate physical frame. However, women leaders, such as Susan B. Anthony, were beginning to make strides in women's rights and opportunities for education and professional practice.

Health practices in the United States before the Civil War were poor. Most physicians of this time were not well educated, and most received their training as apprentices. Sanitation in the cities was poor from the overcrowded conditions.

Civil War

In America, the Civil War (1861 to 1865) gave great impetus to the organization of women and nursing. The need for skilled nurses was increased dramatically, since there were practically no trained nurses in the country. Many women and members of religious groups, without previous training, signed up to serve as nurses, and short intensive courses were given. Even though many women signed up, there were not enough to care for the injured. Lack of supplies, dressings, and drugs to care for the wounded hastened the death of many soldiers. During the war, various women leaders emerged. Clara Barton (1821 to 1912) was one woman recognized for her contribution to care of the soldiers. Dorothea Dix (1803 to 1887) was instrumental in recruiting over 2000 women to serve in the first Nurse Corps of the United States Army. These women were to be over 30 years of age, plain in appearance and dress, and of good moral background. The hours the women worked were long, and many died of the illnesses and diseases they were treating.

Late 1800s

The Civil War raised the consciousness of individuals concerning the role of women as nurses and focused attention on the weakness of a volunteer nursing system. In 1869, a committee of the American Medical Association, headed by Dr. Samuel Gross, conducted a study on the training of nurses. Their findings stated that nursing is as much an art and science as is medicine. The committee recommendations were that (1) every large hospital have a nursing school; (2) local medical agencies establish the schools and the medical staff be responsible for teaching; and (3) that nursing establish societies.

The independent school idea of Florence Nightingale to educate nurses gave way to the hospitals' "training" of nurses. The New England Hospital for Women and Children's Training School for Nurses in Boston was opened in 1872. The "first trained nurse in America" was Linda Richards, who was graduated from this school in 1873. She made many reforms, especially in the area of mental health in America, and instituted the idea of keeping written records on students during their education.

In 1873, three schools of nursing based on the Nightingale plan were opened—Bellevue Training School in New York, Connecticut Training School in New Haven, and the Boston Training School. The practical experience gained while caring for patients was the focus of these schools. The terms "professional school" and "school of higher education" were used synonymously at this time. Mary Eliza Mahoney was the first African-American nursing school graduate. She graduated from the New England Hospital for Women and Children in 1879 (Kalisch & Kalisch, 1995).

Isabel Hampton Robb attended Bellevue Training School and later helped to organize Johns Hopkins Training School. She became its first "principal" in 1889 and is credited with writing the first standardized nursing text in the United States, *Nursing—Its Principles and Practice for Hospital and Private Use*. She was active in organizations that were forerunners of the American Nurses Association. She was also one of the founders of the *American Journal of Nursing*. She thought nursing programs should be 3 years in length instead of the usual one. She also suggested that students should work a maximum of 8 hours a day and receive no payment for their services.

The recommendation of Gross's study for a nursing school in each hospital was not adopted by the many schools that were begun in the late 1800s. The purpose of these schools was switching from educating nurses to supplying student nurses to work for the hospital. The strict application criteria of the Nightingale era, that students were to be of good character and health and have a good education, were disregarded. Hospitals began to admit any person interested in nursing. Hospital administrators found students, in contrast to graduate nurses, worked very cheaply and were easily disciplined. All nurses were expected to be obedient, devoted to duty, and unselfish. Rigid rules were to be followed or the student was dismissed. Curriculums were changed to focus on care of the sick only. No longer were preventive health care and the meeting of psychosocial needs addressed. Students were used primarily to staff the hospital; education was secondary.

Examples of the duties from the floor nurse in 1887 are listed below.

In addition to caring for your 50 patients, each nurse will:

1. Daily sweep and mop the floors of your ward, dust the patient's furniture and windowsills.
2. Maintain an even temperature in your ward by bringing in a scuttle of coal for the day's business.
3. Light is important to observe the patient's condition. Therefore, each day fill kerosene lamps, clean chimneys, and trim wicks. Wash the windows once a week.
4. The nurse's notes are important in aiding the physician's work. Make your pens carefully; you may whittle nibs to your individual taste.
5. Each nurse on day duty will report every day at 7 A.M. and leave at 8 P.M., except on the Sabbath on which day you will be off from 12 noon to 2 P.M.
6. Graduate nurses in good standing with the director of nurses will be given an evening off each week if you go regularly to church.

7. Each nurse shall lay aside from each payday a goodly sum of her earnings for her benefits during her declining years, so that she will not become a burden. For example, if you earn $30.00 a month you should set aside $15.00.
8. Any nurse who smokes, uses liquor in any form, gets her hair done at a beauty shop, or frequents dance halls will give the director of nurses good reason to suspect her worth, intentions, and integrity.
9. The nurse who performs her labors, serves her patients and doctors faithfully and without fault for a period of five years will be given an increase by the hospital administration of five cents a day providing there are no hospital debts that are outstanding (circa 1887, source unknown).

Even though nursing education emphasized hospital-based practice, two nurses, **Lillian Wald** (1867–1940) and Mary Brewster, focused on community-based practice. In 1893, they founded the Henry Street Settlement to improve the conditions of the poor. Settlements of this type were common in England; however, this was the first American settlement and was unique in that nursing care was aimed beyond care of the sick and prevention of disease to include social services and improvement of environmental conditions. This settlement greatly influenced the establishment of the field of public health. Other settlements began in America based on the Henry Street model. Two were founded in Virginia and California in 1900. Wald proposed public health nursing as a Red Cross program in 1908 and taught at the Johns Hopkins School of Nurses. In 1912, Wald became the first president of the then newly formed National Organization for Public Health Nursing. The purpose of this organization was to set up standards for and foster group interest in public health nursing. Wald is considered to be the founder of public health nursing.

Turn of the Century

At the turn of the century, many discoveries in medical science were occurring, and improved aseptic techniques were being relayed to nurses from physicians. Through these discoveries and innovations, nursing focused primarily on technical and psychomotor aspects of care, while the preventive and psychosocial aspects of nursing care were deemphasized. The number of schools of nursing rapidly increased, from 4 in 1873 to over 400 by 1900. With an increase in hospital-based programs came a decrease in emphasis of the nurse's role in nonhospital settings. Many of these schools did not have faculties and used the students to staff the hospitals. They had poorly designed curriculums with sporadic lectures by physicians. Physicians were also realizing the need for skilled hospital nursing and began writing textbooks on nursing techniques and the management of the sick. No longer were nurses teaching the students about nursing. The physicians often focused only on the technical areas. A typical schedule for the students was a $6\frac{1}{2}$-day work week, 10 to 12 hours per day, with duties in the wards, laundry, or kitchen (Fitzpatrick, 1983, p. 69).

The female positions on the governing boards of training schools were being taken over by males. Although other comparable professions such as teaching were taking the more direct route to a system of educational preparation based in institutions of higher learning, nursing failed to follow suit. Society was very willing to support the education of teachers but did not see a need to educate nurses in universities.

Adelaide Nutting (1858 to 1948), a Johns Hopkins graduate, was the first nurse to attend Teachers College, Columbia University, and became the first professor of nursing in the world. She established a 3-year education program for nurses. Nutting was responsible for initiating a course of study in public health nursing as a result of increased student interest in the field of social and preventative work. Utilizing many of Nutting's ideas, Lillian D. Wald introduced a course of study for preparation in public health nursing.

Nutting also studied the hours that student nurses were working (15 hours per day, 105 hours per week) and observed that the students were functioning as servants for the hospital. She made the following recommendations for nursing education: (1) preparatory courses in nursing should be taught in a school outside the hospital; (2) the school should arrange with the hospital for clinical experience for the student; (3) the school should be independent of the hospital; and (4) students should pay tuition (Nutting, 1926, p. 38).

Nutting's recommendations were not followed, since the general feeling in the United States at this time was that nurses were overtrained, even though their education contained a minimal amount of theory. Society thought that nurses were receiving too much theory, which caused them to make inquiries and even question physicians' orders. This was believed to be beyond the scope of the nurse's role. Autonomy of nursing practice espoused by Florence Nightingale was lost but not forgotten. In direct contrast, Lavinia Dock, author of a textbook for nurses, characterized nursing education as "martinet discipline, routinism, and institutionalism," and as "repressing individuality and sending out a set of machines all in the same mold with the same ideas and habits." Physicians have a tendency "to limit and restrict nurses to a strict and literal carrying out of orders and to a technically perfect attendance on themselves," a condition that had gone too far (Stewart, 1944, p. 150).

In the early schools, superintendents of nurses taught the classes. Eventually, physicians taught the nursing classes and wrote the nursing texts. Central themes were developed primarily around medical treatment rather than the role of the nurse in patient care. Perhaps this was due to the fact that nursing education was not in settings that aimed at identifying a body of knowledge, nor were nurses taught research methods by which to determine nursing care. Formal nursing organizations by which nurses could transmit information in a systematic manner or effect change on a large scale were just developing. As nursing evolved, some of the nursing terminology changed. For example, "training" was changed to "education," "superintendent" to "director," and "training school" to "school of nursing" (Dolan, 1983).

Even though the number of diploma programs was increasing, there was some movement to have nursing education in a college setting rather than in a hospital. Through the efforts of Dr. Richard O. Beard, the first school for the basic preparation of nurses within a university setting was started in 1909 at the University of Minnesota. This program combined college courses and nursing education as an integral part of the university. It became recognized as a new type of educational structure for nursing.

World War I

Just prior to World War I, there were trained nurses available to give care for the first time in history. World War I, however, created an increased demand for nurses to care for the wounded. The Army School of Nursing was organized and graduated the first class of nurses in 1921. The purpose of this school was to provide students to care for the sick and wounded in military hospitals. The last class graduated in 1933, and the program was then discontinued for economic reasons. During the period of the war as many as 100 non–university-based nursing schools per year opened, without regard to sound educational practice. Nurses once again returned to the apprenticeship method for training; this stifled any move back to the university. Many students who cared for patients were taught skills, with little or no instruction based on nursing's body of knowledge.

Following World War I, attempts to change the direction of nursing and nursing education were resumed. In 1918, the Rockefeller Foundation formed a committee to study nursing education. Originally, this early landmark study was directed toward the education of public health nurses but later was broadened to include all of nursing education. Findings from this study were published in 1923 in the report *Nursing and Nursing Education in the United States.*

This study is referred to as the **Goldmark Report.** Findings of this study related to nursing education indicated that:

1. Sciences, theory, and practice of nursing were frequently taught by unprepared instructors in poorly equipped basement classrooms.
2. Hospitals controlled the total teaching hours, reduced the ground covered to the barest outline, or might omit some subjects entirely.
3. Lectures were often given to students at night after a hard day's work.
4. Students' practical experience was usually limited to those experiences found in the hospital. The student learned to nurse those patients for whom the hospital cared.
5. The practical experience might be under the supervision of graduate nurses who had neither preparation nor time to teach (Goldmark, 1923, pp. 310–312, cited in Kalisch & Kalisch, 1986, p. 376).

One of the recommendations of the Goldmark Report was that university schools of nursing be developed in an attempt to make the programs independent of hospital needs and to improve nursing education. This was the concept recommended by Florence Nightingale, which had been discarded around the turn of the century. Another recommendation was that a high school education should be required as a minimum prerequisite for entry into schools of nursing. Nursing programs were to include at least 4 months of basic science and the arts of nursing and were to be shortened to 28 months, with work weeks no longer than 40 to 48 hours. Other recommendations were that all instructors should have basic hospital training and that the apprentice system of training be abolished. Though the recommendations for nursing education have received the most emphasis, the Goldmark Report did not neglect its original focus on public health nursing. Among other things, it was concluded that both "bedside nursing care and health teaching for preventative care should be combined in one generalized service as opposed to the separated services and agencies that were more common at the time" (Kelly, 1995, p. 66). As an outcome of the Goldmark Report, the Yale University School of Nursing and the Western Reserve University School of Nursing were opened. Many substandard schools closed, and high school graduation became a prerequisite (Dolan, 1983).

The Goldmark Report did not make a strong impact on nursing education. The news media did not disseminate the information to the general public. The role of women at this time was still to be subservient to male domination, and the schools of nursing were under the control of hospital administrations. Also, physicians were considered in charge of health care and responsible for all related matters. So the social climate for widespread change in nursing and nursing education did not materialize (Matejski, 1981).

The Committee on the Grading of Nursing Schools was organized in 1925. The purpose of this committee was to grade nursing schools and to study the work of nurses in order to define nursing functions. The study lasted 8 years, finishing with two written reports. The first, *Nurses, Patients and Pocketbooks* (1928), looked at the supply and demand of nurses; the other report, *Nursing Schools Today and Tomorrow* (1934), described the number of nursing schools and the type of educational experience they offered. The study identified concerns over the number of schools and their limited curriculums. The overall recommendations of these studies were that nursing adopt a collegiate level of education, enrich the curriculum, and better prepare both student and nurse. The study established specific standards that formed a beginning framework for collegiate education, including the recommendation that faculty members were to have college degrees. The actual grading of nursing schools was not carried out by this committee, because of the wide differences in the nursing programs in America.

The Committee on the Grading of Nursing Schools outlined four tasks:

1. Reduce the number of inferior schools and improve the supply of nurses, which meant raising entrance requirements to admit only qualified students.
2. Replace students with graduate nurses, which would shift patient care responsibility from students to graduates.
3. Help hospitals meet the costs of graduate nurse service so that hospitals could afford to hire qualified nurses.
4. Receive public support for nursing education, allowing nurse educators instead of hospital administrators to assume the role of heads of schools of nursing (Committee on the Grading of Nursing Schools, 1928).

The Committee on the Grading of Nursing Schools studied societal role expectations of the nurse. It was found that the patient expected the nurse to be a provider of comfort, amiability, gentleness, and knowledge. In addition, the physician expected loyalty, obedience, and support of his skill to the patient. The hospital administrator had additional expectations related to sharing the administrative responsibilities in the health care institutions. Finally, the community expected the nurse to be well disciplined, resourceful, and courageous (Committee on the Grading of Nursing Schools, 1934, pp. 79–80).

World War II

In the early 1920s, nursing began to identify more specific educational criteria, which led to the development and opening of more baccalaureate programs within institutions of higher education (e.g., Francis Payne Bolton School of nursing, Western Reserve University, 1923; Yale University, 1924; University of Chicago, 1925). At a time when nursing was emerging as a profession with distinct educational criteria, the health care needs of World War II increased the demand for nurses. World War II did not affect nursing as negatively as had previous wars, because of the increased number of nursing programs, the availability of monies for nursing education, and the strong response of graduate nurses to serve in the army; however, federal monies were needed to help schools of nursing increase their enrollments. The federal government appropriated funds for nursing education in civilian schools. In 1943, the Nurse Training Act, also referred to as the Bolton Act, created the Cadet Nurse Corps and assisted with the education of nurses. This act provided free tuition, fees, uniforms, and stipends for students (Donahue, 1985). The increased availability of monies made it possible for prospective students, those between the ages of 17 and 35, to attend a choice of programs, and the schools were able to improve their programs.

This act increased the number of students enrolled in nursing programs by 30 percent. The number of nurses who actually served in the military was over 76,000. The response to the United States Cadet Nurse Corps program was very positive. By 1948, when the program was terminated, over 125,000 students had graduated.

Both the Army and Navy had nurse corps during the war; however, the corps did not become permanent parts of the armed services until 1947. At this time, Public Law 36 was enacted, which authorized Army nurses to have permanent commissioned status. Prior to this time, nurses in the military only held "relative rank," which did not qualify them for full benefits. In spite of the Army and Navy corps, there was a critical shortage of nurses in America on the battlefield. Thus, in 1945, the President of the United States asked Congress to pass a bill drafting nurses. The nursing organizations lobbied for a bill to include both men and women, not just nurses, as part of the draft. This was discussed by Congress for 3 months but was dropped without passage when the war ended.

It is evident that the recognized societal need for nurses and the regard for nurses as a group has changed greatly since the time of Florence Nightingale. The remainder of this chapter focuses on how nursing education and nursing as a profession continued to develop and change after World War II.

After World War II

The war brought about changes in nursing and nursing education. Curriculums were improved, the clinical experience hours for students were reduced to 48 hours per week, and faculty were better prepared to teach. Shortages of nurses existed and many states developed short, technically oriented programs. These programs had a different educational orientation and level of preparation. The graduates of these programs were vocational, or practical, nurses. The first school was organized in 1897 but did not flourish. From 1947 to 1954 practical schools of nursing developed from 36 to over 260. By the mid 1950s more than 50 percent of nursing personnel were nonprofessionals. Today there are more than 1100 practical nursing programs. The largest numbers of these programs are located in the southern part of the United States. Procedures were instituted for the licensure of practical nurses (LPN) after the mid 1940s. The National Association of Practical Nurse Education, established during the war, was influential in the development of practical nurse programs and practical nurse licensure.

Dr. Esther Lucille Brown, a sociologist, conducted a study on nursing funded by the Carnegie Foundation, called *Nursing for the Future* (**Brown Report**) (1948). This landmark study focused on nursing service and education in terms of what was best for society, not necessarily for the nursing profession. In regard to nursing education, Dr. Brown discovered the need for an educational program with two types of preparation. The first type was to provide a foundation that would permit continuing growth in many aspects: positive health and integration of personality; insight into own motivation, behavior of others, and cultural patterns; ability to use spoken and written language; skill in analyzing problems, obtaining data, and formulating conclusions; perspective gained through historical and anthropological records; understanding of the rights and responsibilities of citizenship; and membership in a profession. The second type of preparation related to technical skills. Dr. Brown cautioned that these skills must be far broader than those traditionally taught in hospital training schools. She thought that only institutions of higher education could provide a base broad enough for such preparation. In terms of nursing service, Dr. Brown recommended mandatory licensure, expansion of in-service education with a focus on interpersonal relationships, improved salaries and professional growth opportunities, development of clinical specialists, and increased research for nursing practice (Brown, 1948).

Nursing continued to grow as a profession in the 1950s. A new type of nursing program was begun in America in 1952 at Teachers College, Columbia University, by **Mildred Montag.** This was the origin of **associate degree** or **community or junior college** programs for nursing. These programs were shorter than the traditional 3-year **diploma** and the 4-year **baccalaureate degree.** Mildred Montag proposed that the graduates of the associate degree programs would be nursing technicians, with nursing functions narrower in scope than those of the professional nurse but broader in scope than those of the practical nurse. These nurses could assist in the planning, implementation, and evaluation of nursing care with supervision (Montag, 1951) (Fig. 3–2).

According to Montag, the curriculum of the associate degree was to be established in a 2-year community or junior college, with clinical experience in a hospital. Graduates could then take the state board licensing examination, the same examination as the diploma and baccalaureate graduates. The associate degree was intended to be a terminal degree because the objectives and program content of this program were different from that of the baccalaureate program. This proposal caused considerable discussion and controversy. Since the proposal was made in 1951, the number of associate degree programs has grown to more than 857 (National League for Nursing, 1993). Montag's original idea for these graduates to be "technical" nurses has not materialized, nor has the degree become a terminal one.

The associate degree nursing program helped to alleviate nursing shortages. Its objectives were not the development of nursing as a profession or the building of a theoretical base for nursing. Therefore, movement toward baccalaureate education with an emphasis on theory building, research, and a conceptual approach to nursing practice was necessary. This need has been identified, from the 1960s

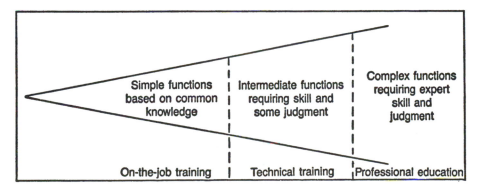

Figure 3–2. The level of nursing responsibility depends on the level of education. *(From Montag, M., p. 4.)*

until the present, in numerous reports whose purpose was assessing services and identifying nursing needs.

The **Surgeon General's Report** in 1963, *Toward Quality in Nursing: Needs and Goals,* placed emphasis on the quality of patient care. A need for increased numbers of nursing schools in colleges and universities was identified to meet this goal. A baccalaureate degree in nursing was recommended for head nurse or team leader positions in hospitals and for nurses in positions outside hospitals. The study also identified areas of society not being represented in nursing, such as men, older women, and minority students, and emphasized the need for research. Advice was requested on the role of the government in providing nursing service. The Nurse Training Act of 1964 provided funds to assist students and schools of nursing in the educative process.

The **American Nurses Association (ANA)** took a stand on nursing education in the **ANA Position Paper** of 1965 (ANA, 1966). This publication took into consideration the rapidly changing health care needs of American society. Technical and scientific changes were occurring faster, causing a need for an increase in the educational level of practitioners in all fields. For nursing to keep pace with these changes and to provide quality nursing, the American Nurses Association stated: "Education for those who work in nursing should take place in institutions of learning within the general system of education" (p. 515). The paper further stated: "Minimal preparation for beginning professional nursing practice at the present time should be the baccalaureate degree education in nursing" and recommended that associate degree education in nursing should be the minimum preparation for beginning technical nursing practice. This paper has caused considerable controversy, which continues today, although there is progress toward meeting these recommendations.

An Abstract for Action (the **Lysaught Report**) (1970) resulted from a national study focusing on the provision of quality patient care, chaired by Jerome Lysaught for the National Commission for the Study of Nursing and Nursing Education. The impetus for this study came from the Surgeon General's 1963 Report. Both nursing and non–nursing members served on this committee. The commission studied various areas of nursing, including:

- Supply and demand for nurses
- Nursing roles and functions
- Nursing education
- Nursing careers

The report included 58 recommendations with the outcome of four major recommendations. It was recommended that research funds be allocated to study nursing's impact on health care and to study nursing education. Many recommendations of this study reinforced the position that nursing education should take place in institutions of higher learning, the same recommendation made by Florence Nightingale over 100 years before and restated in the Goldmark and Brown Reports. It was also recommended that each state form a committee to carry out actions that would ensure nursing education within the mainstream of American educational patterns. Finally, it was suggested that government support be secured for nursing education and research. In 1973, the outcomes of the recommendations of the commission were reported in *From Abstract Into Action*.

The National Commission on Nursing, 1983, was a group of 31 persons from hospital and nursing administration, nursing education, and other related organizations. Its concern was nursing-related problems in health care, especially the supply and demand of nurses and the then-existing shortage of nurses. The five major categories of issues identified by the study include:

1. The status and image of nursing, which includes changes in the nursing role.
2. The interface of nursing education and practice, including models for education to prepare for practice.
3. The effective management of the nursing resource, including such factors as job satisfaction, recruitment, and retention.
4. The relationship among nursing, medical staff, and hospital administration, including nursing's participating in decision-making.
5. The maturing of nursing as a self-determining profession, including defining and determining the nature and scope of practice, the role of nursing leadership, increasing decision making in nursing practice, and the need for unity in the nursing profession (National Commission on Nursing, 1983, p. 5).

The Commission's report supported the trend to upgrade nursing education. Of significance was an emphasis on the development of **graduate education** (**master's** and **doctor's degrees**) programs for nurses.

The National Commission on Nursing Implementation Project (NCNIP) of 1985 followed the Commission on Nursing study and focused on education and credentialing for beginning nursing practice; models for nursing care delivery; and the development of the discipline of nursing. Four prominent nursing organizations (ANA; the American Association of Colleges of Nursing [AACN]; NLN; and the American Organization of Nurse Executives [AONE] were instrumental in this project. The committee requested and was approved for funding from the Kellogg Foundation to implement some of the recommendations from the 1983 studies on nursing from the Institute of Medicine and the National Commission on Nursing Study. Representatives from the nursing organizations listed as well as other nonnursing groups formed a governing body for the project. One outcome of the group was *Nursings' Vital Signs: Shaping the Profession for the 1990s*, which described approaches for education, management and practice research and development.

Other groups have developed resolutions for "entry into practice." The baccalaureate as the entry degree for professional nursing practice is becoming a reality. In 1974, the New York State Nurses' Association passed a resolution that by the year 1985, the baccalaureate in nursing would be the entry level into professional practice. This proposal was also supported by the NLN in 1976. The Ohio Nurses' Association (ONA) developed a similar resolution. In 1985, North Dakota became the first state to set bilevel entry requirements. Beginning in 1987, nurses in North Dakota seeking professional nursing practice were required to have a baccalaureate degree in nursing, and those seeking technical nursing practice must have an associate degree in nursing. By 1992 Maine also required the baccalaureate degree for professional nursing licensure. While the American Nurses Association supported two levels of educational preparation, with the associate degree as the entry level for technical nursing and the baccalaureate degree as the entry level for professional nursing, it also recommended a flexible career ladder approach for nursing education in 1978. A flexible career-ladder approach was also supported by the board of directors of the NLN in 1982.

There continues to be controversy over the concept of a career-ladder approach versus generic baccalaureate education. In 1985, the NLN board of directors passed a resolution supporting baccalaureate education as the entry to professional practice. Some nurse educators support a master's degree in nursing as the first professional degree.

More recently, reports such as the **PEW** continue to make recommendations to chart the course for health and nursing education and practice. In 1995, the PEW Health Professions Commission released the work of the task force on Health Care Workforce Regulation called *Critical Challenges: Revitalizing the Health Professions for the Twenty-First Century* (PEW, 1995). This report acknowledges the changes in health care delivery in the United States and the impact on health care workers. After looking at all health professionals, the Commission recommended a "fundamental alteration of the health professional schools and the ways in which they organize, structure, and frame their programs of education, research, and patient care" (ii). Schools must enlarge the scientific foundation of their programs and include psycho-social-behavioral sciences (p. iii). Specifically for nursing, some of the recommendations include:

- Distinguish between practice responsibilities of these different levels of nursing, focusing associate preparation on the entry level hospital setting and nursing home practice, baccalaureate on hospital-based care management and community-based practice, and master's degree for speciality practice in the hospital and independent practice as a primary care provider.
- Strengthen existing career ladder programs in order to make movement through these levels of nursing as easy as possible (p. vi).
- Reduce the size and number of nursing education programs by 10 percent to 20 percent. These closings should come in associate and diploma degree programs (p. vii).
- Encourage the expansion of the number of master's level nurse practitioner training programs by increasing the level of federal support for students (p. vii).

As a result of the analysis, recommendations, and projections of these many reports, changes have taken place in nursing education. Figure 3–3 illustrates some of the current trends in terms of numbers and types of undergraduate educational programs. As the figure shows, there has been a steady decrease in the number of diploma programs since 1930, following the reports from the Committee on

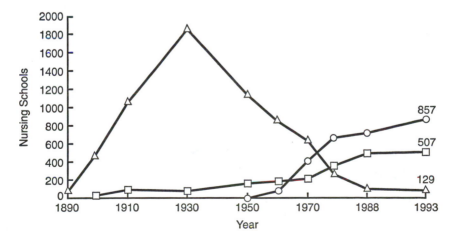

Figure 3–3. Types and numbers of schools of nursing in the United States. △ = Hospital (Diploma), □ = College (Baccalaureate), ○ = College (Associate). *(Compiled from data gathered by the NLN.)*

the Grading of Nursing Schools. Along with this decrease, there has been a gradual increase in numbers of associate and baccalaureate degree programs. This trend began to develop in the 1950s after the Brown Report was released. The number of graduates by types of programs can be seen in Figure 3–4.

Concurrent with the changes in numbers of programs are the changes in numbers of graduates from these programs. While diploma schools graduated 89 percent of nurses in 1955, in 1993 they graduated approximately 8 percent of the registered nurses. In 1993 there were 88,149 graduates from basic nursing programs; 6,937, or 7.8 percent, were from diploma programs; 56,770, or 64 percent, were from associate degree programs; and 24,442, or 28 percent were from baccalaureate programs (NLN, 1995). The distribution of programs providing basic nursing preparation varies from state to state. Figure 3–5 depicts the geographic distribution of nursing programs throughout the United States.

Graduate education programs in nursing, including master's and doctoral preparation, has developed rapidly in the 1980s and 1990s. This is in response to the needs of nurses to be prepared for advanced practice as clinical specialists, administrators, educators, and researchers. Data from the NLN (1995) indicate that from 1985 to 1993 there was a 36 percent increase in enrollment at the master's level. Programs are few in number in comparison with undergraduate programs, but the numbers are increasing.

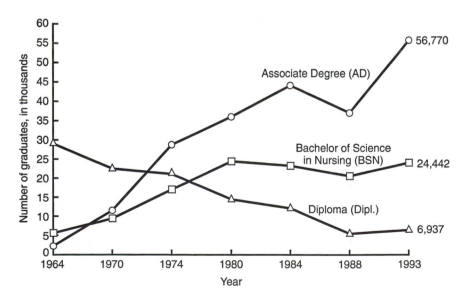

Figure 3–4. Types and numbers of graduates from schools of nursing in the United States. *(Data based on figures from the NLN.)*

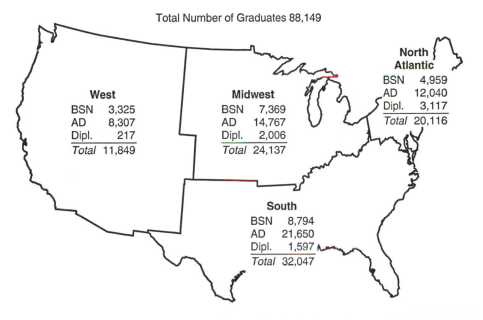

Figure 3–5. Graduations from basic nursing programs throughout the United States. *(Data from Nursing Data Review, 1995.* New York: NLN, 1992–1993.)

The earliest graduate programs in nursing (prior to 1952) were diverse in nature, and many schools considered any course work beyond the diploma to be postgraduate education. Usually the differences between baccalaureate and master's programs were not clarified. The nurse clinician was described as one giving care on an advanced level. In 1953, the newly established **National League for Nursing (NLN)** gave impetus to many nursing educators to formulate and develop programs for master's degrees in nursing. The primary areas of emphasis of these programs were to be research and specialization. In the 1960s, a physician in collaboration with a school of nursing in Colorado began development of the role of a nurse practitioner as one who worked in ambulatory care settings (See Chap. 6). By 1963, 32 master's programs were in operation. The Nurse Training Act of 1964 helped to support further the development of all nursing programs, including master's programs. By the late 1960s, the master's degree in nursing had become widely recognized as important for nurses in leadership positions (Fitzpatrick, 1983). Graduate education is necessary for nursing to advance as a discipline and further develop its own body of knowledge.

Data provided by the **American Association of Colleges of Nursing AACN** (1994) indicate that master's programs continue to increase (328 master's programs in 1994, an increase of 8.7 percent

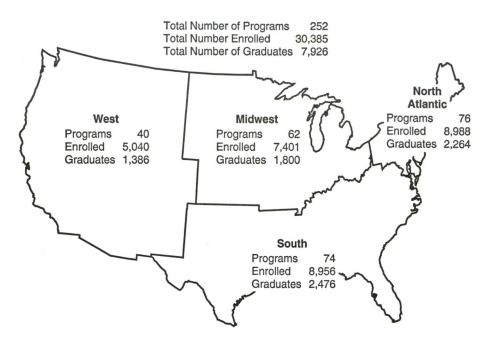

Total Number of Programs   252
Total Number Enrolled   30,385
Total Number of Graduates 7,926

West
Programs   40
Enrolled   5,040
Graduates 1,386

Midwest
Programs   62
Enrolled   7,401
Graduates 1,800

North Atlantic
Programs   76
Enrolled   8,988
Graduates 2,264

South
Programs   74
Enrolled   8,956
Graduates 2,476

Figure 3–6. Graduations from master's nursing programs throughout the United States 1992–1993. *(Data adapted from Nursing Data Review, 1995. New York: NLN, 1995.)*

graduates from the previous year). In 1988, there were 197 master's programs in nursing in the United States, with 5,933 graduates in the same year compared with 6,769 graduates in 1994. Master's education is essential to the development of the practice of nursing. Discussion among nurse educators focuses on the master's level in nursing as the basis for entry into professional practice for the future. Figure 3–6 illustrates the number and distribution of master's nursing programs in the United States.

Doctoral education facilitates nursing's continued development as a discipline and a profession with a theoretical knowledge base validated and expanded by research. The historical development of the doctorate degree in nursing is also unclear. Teachers College at Columbia University established the first doctoral program in 1933, conferring an EdD in nursing. New York University started the first PhD in nursing program in 1934, followed by the University of Pittsburgh in 1954 (Mataruzzo & Abdellah, 1971). Further development of doctoral programs in nursing was slow until the mid-1980s.

H.K. Grace describes some of the difficulty that nursing has faced in the development of doctoral programs:

The evolution of the nursing profession has occurred within a political context that has placed many constraints upon the developmental process. Conflicts within administrative hierarchy, the effects of sexism, and circumscribed roles for women are but a few of the constraints. In this context, doctoral education for nurses and in nursing is but another step in the overall struggle for independence and recognition of worth (1978, p. 114).

During the mid-1980s, there was an increased emphasis on nursing theory and research, which provided impetus for the development of doctoral programs in nursing. By 1993, there were 54 doctoral programs, with several other universities considering the establishment of a program. These 54 programs awarded 381 doctorates, a 25 percent increase over 1988 (NLN, 1995). Between 1983 and 1993, 2,917 doctorates were awarded in nursing. AACN (1994) data indicate a continuing increase in the growth of doctoral programs. The 1993–1994 survey indicates 59 reported doctoral programs, an increase of five from the previous year with an additional 11 programs planned for the future. Graduations in the same years increased from 374 to 380, a 1.6 percent increase for the same years. As doctoral education continues to develop, content and structure of master's programs in nursing will also change. Figure 3–7 illustrates the numbers and graduates from doctoral programs.

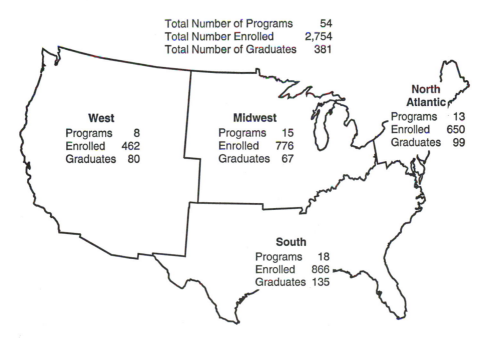

Total Number of Programs   54
Total Number Enrolled   2,754
Total Number of Graduates   381

West
Programs   8
Enrolled   462
Graduates   80

Midwest
Programs   15
Enrolled   776
Graduates   67

North Atlantic
Programs   13
Enrolled   650
Graduates   99

South
Programs   18
Enrolled   866
Graduates   135

Figure 3–7. Graduations from doctoral nursing programs throughout the United States 1992–1993. *(Data adapted from Nursing Data Review, 1995. New York: NLN, 1995.)*

BASIC NURSING EDUCATION

Three types of basic educational programs prepare students to take the licensing examination to qualify as a registered nurse: diploma, baccalaureate, and associate degree. The earliest type is the diploma school program, traditionally in a hospital setting, conferring a diploma of nursing after graduation, and generally lasting 27 to 33 months. An academic degree is not awarded, that is, no college credits. The trend is away from diploma education. Many diploma programs, however, have affiliated with colleges or universities for non-nursing courses such as the social sciences and physical sciences and, to a more limited degree the liberal arts. In many instances existing diploma schools are transferring into developing or already existing associate or baccalaureate degree programs.

Next is the baccalaureate degree program in a college or university, which confers a bachelors' degree after 4 or 5 years of study. These programs traditionally offer clinical experiences in hospital and nonhospital settings and, in particular, community health settings. They offer a broad educational base in arts, humanities, sciences, and nursing, thus providing a framework for students to synthesize and apply knowledge of various disciplines. Students assess, plan, and evaluate care for individuals and groups of clients. Graduates have a beginning understanding of the research process and how nursing functions within society. Baccalaureate programs provide a foundation for graduate study.

The latest type of program to develop is the associate degree program found in community and junior colleges. This program leads to an associate degree in nursing and is 2 academic years in length. The associate degree program traditionally focuses on the individual client and direct patient care. The cultural focus within the curriculum is on the surrounding community and the nurse's response to it. Graduates work in established health care facilities that have well-defined, organized structures, not in independent and community settings (NLN, 1978).

The associate degree program can be described as preparing a technical nurse and the baccalaureate degree program as preparing the professional nurse. The technical nurse can be described as caring for individuals with well-defined health problems and predictable outcomes, whereas the professional nurse *coordinates* and *manages* care of a variety of clients as well as providing care. The knowledge base of the technically prepared nurse includes a circumscribed body of established skills relevant to patient needs, whereas the professional nurse incorporates theory from other disciplines as well as nursing theory in addressing health care needs treated by nursing. The associate-degreed nurse primarily organizes the individual care of clients.

Considerable discussion focuses on what constitutes professional nursing education. Nursing leaders advocate the baccalaureate degree in nursing as the entry level for professional nursing. As previously mentioned, in 1965, the ANA's Position Paper endorsed the position that all nurses be educated in colleges and universities and that the minimum preparation for professional practice be the baccalaureate degree (ANA, 1966).

In 1982, NLN also supported the baccalaureate in nursing as the minimum requirement for professional nursing practice (NLN, 1982). More recently, the ANA Cabinet on Nursing Education submitted a proposed timetable for nursing education preparation to the ANA House of Delegates. This proposal stated that by 1995, 100 percent of the states will have established the ANA standard of the baccalaureate for professional practice, "with the ultimate goal being congruence of professional nurse licensure with the educational base of the baccalaureate in nursing" (ANA Convention, 1984, p. 7). In further support of the baccalaureate in nursing as the first professional degree in nursing, Rogers (1985) stated:

> The distinguishing characteristic of professional education in nursing is the transmission of nursing's body of abstract knowledge, arrived at by scientific research and logical analysis—not a body of technical skills. This is not to deny the importance of technical skills but rather to make clear that it is nursing's organized body of theoretical knowledge that identifies nursing as a profession. It is the utilization of this knowledge in service to people that determines the nature of nursing services. It is this body of knowledge that encompasses nursing's descriptive, explanatory, and predictive principles, principles that guide its practitioners and make possible professional practice (p. 381).

In addition to the need for nurses with master's and doctoral degrees is the growing need for advanced practice nurses—clinical nurses specialists, nurse practitioners, nurse midwives, and nurse anesthetists—to care for patients in all areas of the health care delivery system. In nursing, most master's programs (generally 1 or 2 years in length) have theoretical and clinical components. The theoretical component focuses on the discipline of nursing and the content of a speciality within the discipline. The clinical components focus on advanced practice skills and on understanding, using, and conducting selected aspects of research. In addition, further role development related to advanced practice is facilitated, and the social, political, ethical, legal, and economic factors influencing health care delivery, its delivery system, and nursing are emphasized. There is movement toward recognition by national certifying bodies of advanced practice that will require a master's degree. Also available are master's degrees in nursing programs that focus on education as well as development of advanced practice skills. Programs preparing nurse administrators are also offered at the master's level. Often these are dual-degree programs such as the MSN/MBA (master's of science in nursing/master's in business administration) or the MSN/MPA (master's of science in nursing/master's in public administration).

Doctoral programs in nursing often prepare the graduate for the advancement of the discipline and profession of nursing through the preparation of the nurse researcher. These programs also prepare nurse educators, who must have the doctorate for tenure and academic advancement in colleges and universities. They contribute to the development of the nurse leader for top-level positions in a variety of health care arenas focusing on public policy and nursing policy related to health care and the health care delivery system. Various doctoral degrees are awarded, including the doctor of philosophy (PhD), doctor of nursing science (DNSc), doctor of science in nursing (DSN), doctor of nursing education (DNEd), doctor of education (EdD), and doctor of public health (DPH).

SOCIALIZATION AND EDUCATIONAL PREPARATION

The process of education for a profession focuses on adult learners who bring with them to their course work a sense of purpose and self-direction. The nursing curriculum is designed to assist the student in the process of socialization into the discipline and profession of nursing. Students are assisted in learning the theory, facts, and skills necessary for the practice of nursing as well as internalizing the professional culture. The curriculum also has another important focus, personal development.

The curriculum of each school is developed from the faculty's philosophy or belief about nursing. The usual components of a philosophy are beliefs about the person, health, environment, education, and nursing. From these beliefs an outline, or conceptual framework, is developed, which then determines the curriculum plan and the goals each student is expected to achieve by graduation. This framework provides the basis for the student's personal and professional growth. School catalogues contain statements of the philosophy and the goals to be achieved by the graduate. New students may find it helpful to review the catalogues for this framework.

Incorporated into the nursing curriculums are principles of adult education. *Androgogy* has been described by Knowles (1968) as the art or science of helping adults to learn. The major purpose of the process of adult education is to help adults achieve their full potential. Some principles of adult education that are incorporated into the curriculum may include recognizing the students' motivation and self-direction; providing learning experiences that build on previous knowledge; incorporating what the students want to learn about the profession; and participating in a variety of experiences with feedback on their progress for competency development.

The curriculum also includes liberal arts and humanities courses to familiarize the student with cultural differences, assist in personal growth, and create an educational base on which to build nursing knowledge. Most nursing curriculums are designed to move from simple to more complex ideas. For instance, the study of an individual person is less complex than the study of several people interacting in groups or within societies. Curriculums also are based on concepts composed of facts, theories, research findings, and principles. A problem-solving method, such as that provided by the nursing process, is integral to the curriculum. Basic concepts can be applied in many situations. An example of this is wound healing. The principle of asepsis (the absence of disease-producing organisms) and the facts involved in the process of wound healing are introduced to students. These are two of the facts and principles that make up the concept of wound healing. Wounds resulting from a surgical incision (e.g., removal of the appendix), a traumatic injury (e.g., cuts, bruises, and fractures from an automobile accident), or a disease process (e.g., heart attack) all undergo the same healing process. The location and nature of the injury may vary, but the concept remains the same and can be applied in each situation. As more complex concepts are introduced, they begin to form a pattern, with each concept building on the other. For instance, stress, a complex concept, may slow the healing process; thus, the two concepts of stress and wound healing interrelate to form a pattern.

CRITICAL THINKING

Current emphasis is being placed in nursing curriculums on the **critical thinking** process as a basis for patient nursing care decisions as well as understanding and functioning within the health care delivery system and the profession of nursing. Bandman & Bandman (1995) state that "to think critically is to examine assumptions, beliefs, propositions, and the meaning and uses of words, statements, and arguments." It defines "the conditions under which sound and valid conclusions are drawn (p. 4). Bandman & Bandman provide a checklist of critical thinking functions in nursing (p. 7):

1. Use the processes of critical thinking in all of daily living.
2. Discriminate among the uses and misuses of language in nursing.

3. Identify and formulate nursing problems.
4. Analyze meanings of terms in relation to their indication, their cause or purpose, and their significance.
5. Analyze arguments and issues into premises and conclusions.
6. Examine nursing assumptions.
7. Report data and clues accurately.
8. Make and check inferences based on data, making sure that the inferences are at least plausible.
9. Formulate and clarify beliefs.
10. Verify, corroborate, and justify claims, beliefs, conclusions, decisions, and actions.
11. Give relevant reasons for beliefs and conclusions.
12. Formulate and clarify value judgments.
13. Seek reasons, criteria, and principles that effectively justify value judgments.
14. Evaluate the soundness of conclusions.

Curriculum design (e.g., eclectic, slope, integrated) is based on the philosophy of the school and each approach presents the theory and skills of nursing in a different manner. Common to all curriculums is content related to the professional development and trends in nursing. Two approaches, *integrated* and *traditional,* are frequently seen as models for nursing curriculums. A brief description of these two approaches follows.

The Integrated Approach

The integrated approach is organized around general processes such as growth and development or psychological and physiological processes. For example, the integrated approach may be used in studying fluid and electrolyte balance for a person of any age, condition, or classification. A person having surgery, a pregnant mother, a child with a burn, or a diabetic may all be experiencing some alteration in fluid balance. These clients are studied together in relation to fluid balance, and this alteration is the integrating process.

The Traditional Approach

The traditional approach is organized around client care classifications, currently organized into psychiatric and mental health, care of the adult, emerging family, care of children, and community health nursing. Within many traditionally organized programs, threads or integrating concepts are identified and run throughout the curriculum as unifying components. Using our example, fluid and electrolyte balance is studied in relation to adults, children, and pregnant women. Thus, fluid and electrolyte balance becomes an integrated concept within each course.

Formerly, state board of nursing examinations were based on medical, surgical, pediatric, psychiatric, and obstetrical nursing. Today the examinations use an integrated approach based on nursing process. Using this decision-making process, the focus is on individuals, families, and groups. Consideration is given to the autonomy of the client in making decisions. (See Chapter 8.)

CURRENT STATUS OF THEMES AND ISSUES IN NURSING

The issues and trends evident throughout nursing history still affect nursing today. The religious domination felt during the early periods in nursing is now transformed into the spiritual aspect of care that can span many cultures and beliefs. The influence of the military is still perceptible in areas such as structure of organizations, uniforms, and time schedules. Wars have contributed to advances in health care and methods of dealing with the sick and injured. Triage, early ambulation after surgery, and trauma care are all outcomes of caring for the wounded. Knowledge explosion in areas of science and technology continues to challenge nursing to develop new and innovative ways to provide care to clients and yet be cost conscious. In recent decades, computers have influenced every aspect of our daily lives. Computers provide vast capacities for data storage, handling, and manipulation. Nurses use computers for several purposes including client care management, client record maintenance, staffing patterns, budgeting, literature searches, statistical analysis, word processing, and education, as in computer-aided instruction.

The equal rights movement has influenced women's image in society. This is seen in the number of women in the work force and with sexism being removed from textbooks, television, and other forms of communication. More men have entered the profession; nurses are forming unions for better working conditions and wages; more women are in leadership positions; and nursing has expanded into independent practice and other autonomous positions. These changes have affected the way women in nursing view themselves, their profession, and their positions. Changes in opportunities for women, not just in nursing but in other professions, have impacted on the growing need for nurses in various areas of practice. Nurses are responding to the nursing shortage by being actively involved politically and economically to improve the consumer's view of nursing and recruit more people into nursing.

Nurses are just beginning to expand their positions, assert themselves in terms of their knowledge and skill levels, and become aware of all they have to offer in addressing health care needs. The contemporary nurse is a forward-thinking decision maker who is an initiator of change.

SUMMARY

Nursing has moved from the traditional cure orientation to one of health promotion and health maintenance. Nursing no longer views the client solely in terms of illness care. The development of the discipline of nursing has progressed from the untrained ministering of matrons and "nurses" of early civilizations to the education of professional nurses in modern facilities. Florence Nightingale was an initiator in leading nursing toward modern professional status. It is evidence that nursing is integrally involved in social change. The needs of the military and wars significantly influenced the direction of nursing and nursing education. Expanding knowledge in science and technology, with emphasis on hospital care, caused nursing practice and nursing education to be associated with hospitals. Health needs of those outside the hospital, however, continue to elicit a response from nursing in terms of practice and educational preparation.

Movement toward the education of nurses in colleges and universities has permitted the formation of a body of nursing knowledge and the learning of nursing research skills. Through the use of that knowledge and those skills, nursing can continue to grow and evaluate its own progress. It is projected that the change in the educational preparation of nurses will effect a change in the area of nursing practice and practice issues.

▸ Questions for Discussion

1. Compare and contrast nursing education in the past with present educational trends.
2. During Florence Nightingale's time, nurses were considered to be of very low social class and moral character. How do you think nurses are viewed by society today?
3. After reading about the development of nursing, formulate some of your ideas about the future of nursing. What changes do you see currently being made?
4. What effect has the historical role of women exerted on the development of nursing?
5. Discuss the influence Florence Nightingale had on the development of schools of nursing.

6. Describe the impact the Henry Street Settlement had on community health.
7. Describe social issues and their impact on nursing and nursing education.
8. What impact did the ANA Position Paper, Goldmark Report, Brown Report, and Lysaught Report have on nursing and nursing education?

REFERENCES

American Association of Colleges of Nursing. *1993–1994 Enrollments and Graduations in Baccalaureate and Master's Programs in Nursing* (Publication #9394-1). Washington, D.C.: AACN; 1994.

American Nurses Association's first position on education for nursing. *Am J Nurs.* 1966; 66:515.

Bandman E, Bandman B. *Critical Thinking in Nursing.* 3rd ed. Norwalk, CT: Appleton & Lange; 1995.

Brown E. *Nursing for the Future.* New York: Russell Sage Foundation; 1948.

Bullough V, Bullough B. *History, Trends, and Politics of Nursing.* Norwalk, CT: Appleton-Century-Crofts; 1984.

Committee on the Grading of Nursing Schools. *Nurses, Patients and Pocketbooks.* New York: National League for Nursing Education; 1928.

Committee on the Grading of Nursing Schools. *Nursing Schools Today and Tomorrow.* New York: National League for Nursing Education; 1934.

Dickens C. *Martin Chuzzlewit.* Boston: Estes and Lauriat; 1896.

Dolan J. *Nursing in Society, A Historical Perspective.* 15th ed. Philadelphia: Saunders; 1983.

Donahue PM. *Nursing, the Finest Art.* St. Louis: Mosby; 1985.

Fitzpatrick M. *Prologue to Professionalism.* Bowie, MD: Brady Communications; 1983.

Goldmark J. *Nursing and Nursing Education in the United States.* New York: Macmillan; 1923.

Grace HK. The development of doctoral education in nursing: A historical perspective. In: Chaska NL, ed. *The Nursing Professional: Views Through the Mist.* New York: McGraw-Hill; 1978.

Jenson D, Spaulding J, Cody E. *History and Trends of Professional Nursing.* 4th ed. St. Louis: Mosby; 1955.

Kalisch P, Kalisch B. *The Advances of American-Nursing.* 3rd ed. Philadelphia: Lippincott; 1995.

Kelly L. *Dimensions of Professional Nursing.* 7th ed. New York: McGraw-Hill; 1995.

Knowles M. Andragogy, not pedagogy. *Adult Leadership.* 1968; 16:350–386.

Lysaught J. *An Abstract for Action.* New York: McGraw-Hill; 1970.

Mataruzzo J, Abdellah F. Doctoral education for nurses in the United States. *Nurs Res.* 1971; 20:404–414.

Matejski M. Nursing education, professionalism and autonomy: Social constraints and the Goldmark Report. *Adv Nurs Sci.* 1981; 4:17–30.

Montag M. *The Education of Nursing Technicians.* New York: Putnam; 1951.

National Commission on Nursing. *Summary report and recommendations.* Chicago: The Commission; 1983.

National League for Nursing. *Competencies of associate degree education in nursing.* (Publication #23–1731) Council of Associate Degree Programs. NY: NLN; 1978.

National League for Nursing. *Nursing Data Review, 1995.* (Publication #19–2686) New York. NLN; 1995.

Nightingale F. *Notes on Nursing.* New York: Appleton-Century-Crofts; 1940.

Notter L, Spalding E. *Professional Nursing, Foundations, Perspectives, Relationship.* 9th ed. Philadelphia: Lippincott; 1976.

Nutting A. *A Sound Basis for Schools of Nursing.* New York: Putnam; 1926.

PEW Health Professions Commission. *Critical Challenges: Revitalizing the Health Professions for the Twenty-First Century.* Third Report of the PEW Health Professions Commission; 1995.

Rogers M. The nature and characteristics of professional education for nursing. *J Prof Nurs.* 1985; 1:381–383.

Stewart I. *The Education of Nurses. Historical Foundations and Modern Trends.* New York: Macmillan; 1944.

BIBLIOGRAPHY

Dock L, Stewart I. A *Short History of Nursing.* 4th ed. New York: Putnam; 1938.

Forni P. Models for doctoral programs. *Nurs Health Care.* 1989; 10:429–434.

Gaynon D. The first restructuring of American nursing education 1880–1946. *Nurse Educ.* 1985; 10(5):27–31.

Gross S. *Report of Committee on the Training of Nurses.* Transactions of the American Medical Association. Philadelphia: Collins; 1989.

Kalisch B, Kalisch P. Slaves, servants or saints? *Nurs Forum.* 1975; 14:222–263.

Kalisch P, Kalisch B. The image of the nurse in motion pictures. *Am J Nurs.* 1982; 82:605–611.

Kalisch P, Kalisch B. The image of nurses in novels. *Am J Nurs.* 1982; 82:1220–1224.

Kalisch P, Kalisch B. Nurses on prime time television. *Am J Nurs.* 1982; 82:264–270.

McBride AB. Nursing and the women's movement [editorial]. *Image.* 1984; 16(3):66.

Oermann M, Jamison M. Nursing education component in master's programs. *J Nurs Educ.* 1989; 28:252–255.

Seymer L. One hundred years ago. *Am J Nurs.* 1960; 60:658–661.

Smith F. Florence Nightingale. Early feminist. *Am J Nurs.* 1981; 81:1021–1024.

Snyder-Halpern R. Doctoral programs in nursing: An examination of curriculum similarities and differences. *J Nurs Educ.* 1986; 25:358–365.

The role of a nurse in 1887. *Nurs Forum.* 1971; 10:31.

Wakefield-Fisher M, Wright M, Kraft L. A first for the nation: North Dakota and entry into nursing practice. *Nurs Health Care.* 1986; 7:135–141.

Watson J. The evolution of nursing education in the United States: 100 years of a profession for women. *J Nurs Educ.* 1977; 16:31–37.

4

CHAPTER

Socialization and Professional Development

▸ **Questions to think about before reading the chapter**

- Do you think that nursing is viewed as a profession by society and the health care system?
- What components are important when considering a profession?
- How would you describe the role of the nurse?
- What has influenced your idea of a nurse?
- What student learning experiences do you think will prepare you to be a nurse?

▸ **Terms to know**

American Nurses Association (ANA)

American Nurses Association-Political
    Action Committee (ANA-PAC)

Autonomy

International Council of Nurses (ICN)

National League for Nursing (NLN)

National Student Nurses' Association (NSNA)

Profession

Professional

Professional culture

Role development   Socialization

Sigma Theta Tau (STT)

▶ *Introduction*

In the preceding chapters, information was presented concerning the discipline of nursing, the foundations of the profession, and its historical evolution. Study of the historical evolution of nursing reveals that there has begun to emerge a body of knowledge that is guiding the practice of nursing and development of the role of the nurse. Nursing discipline (nursing knowledge) is the basis of practice and has a reciprocal relationship with research. Nursing is a developing profession. The first purpose of this chapter is to examine nursing as a profession using commonly recognized criteria. The second purpose is to introduce the concept of role development and socialization into the discipline and profession of nursing. Finally, a brief overview of political implications is given.

THE PROCESS OF PROFESSIONALIZATION

The term **professional** may bring different images to mind. These images are related to a person's experience. Some may perceive *professional* in terms of a clean, polished business person or a crisp, starched, white-uniformed nurse. To others, *professional* is the opposite of *amateur*. In sports, for example, *professional* implies reimbursement for services, whereas an amateur receives no reimbursement. Members of the three traditional professions, law, medicine, and ministry, have been viewed by others as professionals. None of these definitions is adequate, however, when one is considering nursing as a profession. The professional status of nursing has become a pressing issue for today's nurse.

In retrospect, patterns can be identified in developing professions (the process of professionalization). First, there is a need that is identified by society. Historically, specializations have arisen in response to the identified needs of society. From this response, fundamental skills and knowledge bases are identified by trained personnel and are handed down in an apprenticeship system. In an apprenticeship, information is transmitted, in informal settings such as homes and monasteries, by one considered knowledgeable to those less knowledgeable in the subject. Educational programs, on the other hand, are developed to formalize the transmission of knowledge and to teach more clearly defined theory and skills. Practitioners are educated through this formal process, and payment for services is provided. Formal rules of practice (codes) are devised and enforced by the practitioners. The methods for enforcement of these codes are established by the professional group. In the process of professionalization a group consciousness develops (Guinee, 1970).

The historical development of the discipline of nursing and nursing as a profession reflects the same patterns. Since pre-Christian times, society has identified health care needs. Those of nurturing and caring very early became identified with nursing. From this base, nursing has broadened and expanded its components and related skills so that nursing is involved with the entire response of the person to his or her health state. The early training of nurses was accomplished through apprentice-type education, with knowledge passed on by word of mouth. It was through Florence Nightingale's influence that the educational process for nursing became formalized and the beginning concepts of a theoretical base were established. As a group consciousness arose, nurses began to organize into professional organizations such as the American Nurses Association.

Through professional organizations, a code of nursing and standards of practice were developed. The profession continues to develop means of enforcing these standards. Figure 4–1 illustrates the patterns in the development of professions and disciplines to meet identified health care needs of persons in global interaction

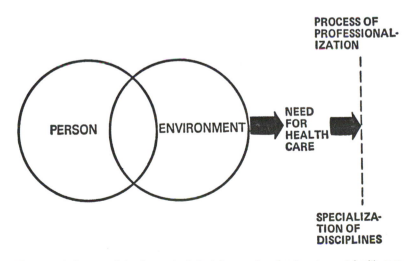

Figure 4–1. Pattern of development of disciplines and professions to meet health care needs.

with the environment. Having evolved through the process of professionalization, a system achieves status as a profession meeting established criteria.

CRITERIA OF A PROFESSION

Around the turn of the 20th century, professionalism was a topic of emphasis and priority in occupational circles. Abraham Flexner (1915) identified areas needing attention in the medical profession and, at the same time, developed criteria for a **profession.** These criteria were applicable to many different professional areas, such as social work, nursing, and medicine. The following are six characteristics of professional activity listed by Flexner (1915, pp. 578–581):

1. It is basically intellectual, carrying with it high individual responsibility.
2. It is learned in nature, because it is based on a body of knowledge.
3. It is basically practical rather than theoretical.
4. Its technique can be taught through educational discipline.
5. It is well organized internally.
6. It is motivated by public interest and altruism.

Since Esther Lucille Brown (1948) identified the confusion in nursing related to meeting professional criteria, nurses and non–nurses have more consciously addressed the issues related to professionalism. Nurses are examining nursing according to the professional criteria to determine its standing as a profession. Characteristics frequently cited in the literature today include those listed by Ellis and Hartley (1995, p. 10)

- Possess a well-defined and well-organized body of knowledge that is on an intellectual level and can be applied to the activities of the group.
- Enlarge a systematic body of knowledge and improve education and service through use of the scientific method.
- Educate its practitioners in institutions of higher education.
- Function autonomously in the formulation of professional control of professional activity.
- Develop within the group a code of ethics.
- Attract to the profession individuals who recognize this occupation as their life work and who desire to contribute to the good of society through service to others.
- Strive to compensate its practitioners by providing autonomy, continuous professional development, and economic security.

In comparing these characteristics, one finds that nursing has already met many of the criteria and is rapidly moving toward meeting them all. Nursing continues to fulfill the initial service needs of society for caring and nurturing. Broadening its initial services to include assisting individuals in promotion and maintenance of health meets current needs of health and society. At present, nursing draws from an evolving body of knowledge involving the arts and sciences. With increasing research and theory development, nursing knowledge continues to be more clearly defined and expanded in scope.

Nursing has its own techniques or skills, which are evident in its areas of expertise. In large part, nursing process has become the cognitive process and the base for defining, planning, implementing, and evaluating nursing care. When a nursing process framework is used, rationale is provided for actions and evaluation occurs, ensuring individual responsibility for these actions. Nursing leaders have identified the need for nursing education to occur within institutions of higher learning, with an emphasis on theory and research as well as practice.

Organizations have been formed within nursing to establish and control policies and activities that are continually incorporated in nursing practice and protected through the legal structure. Because of the social nature of nursing, however, these policies and activities are challenged continually by other societal forces: the bureaucratic hospital, health care system, and professional bodies such as the American Medical Association.

Essential to the establishment of its own policies and activities are the concepts of **autonomy**, individual responsibility, and individual and group accountability. As nursing becomes more clearly defined as a discipline, these concepts as they relate to nursing are more fully developed. The forming of nursing organizations formalized the movement toward autonomy, individual responsibility, and accountability for nursing practice separate from other types of practice, and professional licensure helped continue it. Peer review by nurses has also become a significant issue in terms of nursing autonomy. Independent decisions regarding nursing actions within formal health care institutions and those by the many nurses entering independent practice areas have increased autonomy of nurses. With increased emphasis on health promotion and maintenance and shortened hospital stays, community and home health care is increasing. Nursing continues to focus attention on attracting individuals whose primary motivation is service.

Many factors have enhanced the development of professionalization of nursing. Several of these factors, such as increasing educational standards, increased efforts toward the development of nursing's knowledge base, emphasis on conducting nursing research, and the women's movement, are discussed throughout this book.

Nursing continues to advance in addressing the needs of individuals within society for improvement of health. Nursing is establishing itself as a profession with the development of theories and research, the development of nursing organizations and increased autonomy, and the development of commitment and increased sense of responsibility. Nursing is a growing, developing, and thriving profession in today's society.

NURSING ORGANIZATIONS

An integral part of the development of nursing as a profession was the formation of professional organizations to establish and control policies and activities of nursing practice, and to ensure that progression toward meeting criteria for the profession be maintained. Every profession has an organization composed of its practitioners. The **American Nurses Association (ANA)** is the organization for professional nursing. The ANA was begun in 1896 as the Nurses Associated Alumni of the United States and Canada. In 1911, its name was changed to American Nurses' Association. Its purposes are to foster high standards of nursing practices, promote professional and educational advancement of nurses and promote the welfare of nurses to the end that all people have better nursing care (ANA, 1970).

The ANA provides a foundation for nurses' professional development, establishes standards of practice and codes of ethics, has developed a mechanism for credentialling in a variety of areas, and provides direction for the advancement of nursing practice. It is also active in labor relations and is actively involved in economic and employment issues. Membership in the ANA is open only to registered nurses. It is a formal means of communication for nurses and publishes the *American Journal of Nursing* (AJN). The ANA is a member of the **International Council of Nurses (ICN)** which includes pursing organizations throughout the world. Most states have an organized constituent group of the ANA, which allows for more local control of nursing policies and statewide support for nursing practice. (See Appendix A for listing of state nursing organizations.) Local control and active involvement are enhanced by the organization of districts within each state.

The **National Student Nurses' Association (NSNA)** was created in 1952 with the ANA as a means of professional development for nursing students and for direct participation by students in nursing's development. This association has helped to improve student living conditions and social life within nursing schools. It also has encouraged nursing students to become interested in and aware of current nursing issues and trends. Membership in NSNA is available through many schools of nursing.

Other organizations have been formed to assist in the maintenance of the purposes and goals of professional nursing within the broader perspectives of health care. The best-known example is the **National League for Nursing (NLN),** whose membership comprises nurses, other health care professionals, and community members. The NLN was organized in 1952 to promote the improvement of nursing service and nursing education. One of its major services is accreditation of nursing schools on a voluntary basis, ensuring higher standards for schools of nursing. It also accredits community health agencies. The NLN publishes a list of these accredited programs.

Sigma Theta Tau (STT), the International Nursing Honors Organization, is another organization whose membership is constituted of professional nurses and whose goals focus on quality nursing care, development of the discipline, scholarly activity, and research. Membership is selective and based on guidelines of scholarship.

Specialty organizations have been established to promote specific areas such as practice, education, and administration. The specialty groups offer continuing education, publications, and colleagueship to help nurses remain informed of new advancements and techniques within their areas. Some of these specialty groups include , the Association of Women's Health, Obstetrical and Neonatal Nurses (AWHONN) the American Association of Critical–Care Nurses (AACN), the Association of Occupational Health Nurses (AOHN), the Association of Operating Room Nurses (AORN), the Emergency Department Nurses Association (EDNA), and the American Association of Nurse Anesthetists (AANA). (See Appendix B for listing of specialty groups.)

SOCIALIZATION AND ROLE DEVELOPMENT IN NURSING

Many persons doubtless decide to enter nursing on the basis of predetermined ideas about nursing and the types of jobs and activities nurses perform. These ideas may have been formed from books, the media, and association with health care professionals. Or, they may relate to perceived advantages of nursing such as employment stability, flexibility, diversity, and opportunity.

The Cherry Ames nursing books illustrate how novels can influence the reader's view of a profession. This series of novels was published in the 1940s in an effort to attract more women into the profession (Holt, 1977). These books represented nurses as kind and tolerant women who had high ideals of nursing and service and always followed the physician's orders without question. This image has survived and remains a commonly held view of nurses today. The media help to shape many attitudes about nursing and health care. The public's view of nursing has been directly influenced by the image of nursing on television, in books, and in motion pictures. Kalisch & Kalisch (1982a, b, c) surveyed the media and its portrayal of nursing and found the portrayal adversely affects the nursing profession and its autonomy. Although the media continue to perpetuate the male physician dominance, many television shows are beginning to incorporate the nurse as a team member who has collaborating relationships with other health care professionals. The awareness of nurses as to nursing image has also been heightened so that collective action is being taken to influence the media in accurately portraying nursing and reflecting nursing's involvement in the health care delivery system.

The Student's Experience

Socialization is part of the education that develops the professional ideals and nursing student's norms. Socialization into a profession usually follows a typical pattern. Initially, students bring to their courses of study personal ideas and beliefs about the profession. There are many professionals, whether they are inside or outside of the nursing profession, with whom the students interact. These professionals influence the ideals of the students and contribute to the socialization process. The student internalizes the values of the profession. This whole process is not an easy one, since nursing students have varying concepts of nursing, among themselves and in comparison with faculty views.

As students learn about nursing from experienced professional nurses, their ideas about nursing and the professional image of a nurse will change. Part of the educational process is discussing these ideas with fellow students and faculty and arriving at a common basis of understanding. Nursing curriculums are designed to present new concepts and challenge the old ideas about health, wellness, illness, and caring for clients. This reevaluation is often referred to as **role development** or professional **socialization.**

Socialization is a process or set of activities a person uses to gain knowledge, skills, and behaviors in order to participate as a member of a particular group. Socialization involves a change in values, attitudes, knowledge, and skills. In adults, part of this socialization process includes a desire to learn new roles and related behaviors, building new knowledge from previous learning, having realistic expectations of the educational process, and learning how to deal with new and different role expectations (Brim & Wheeler, 1966). Professional socialization has been further described by Jacox (1973) as gaining an occupational identity and internalizing the values and norms of that profession. Every profession has a specific body of knowledge, values, and skills that set it apart from other professions. The course of study in nursing programs is designed to teach these foundations of the discipline and profession of nursing. By the end of a program, the student will have gained an identity in nursing, will have internalized the values and norms of the profession, and will be equipped with a process for continued learning and accommodation to changing ideas and knowledge.

Cohen (1981) describes four goals of professional socialization. One goal is the learning of theory, facts, and skills. Nursing curriculums incorporate the learning of theory, facts, and skills. **Professional culture** is the internalization of the "values, norms, motivational attributes, and ethical standards held in common by other members of the profession" (Cohen, 1981, p. 15). This professional culture is derived from the interaction of students, faculty, and other health care professionals. Once the culture is internalized, it can be used in situations where there are differing values and attitudes. The last two goals identified by Cohen are the development of a personally and professionally acceptable role, and integrating this role into daily life. These last two goals can be viewed as professional identity, or how the individual wants to be seen by others. These four goals are dynamic and ever-changing and challenge the professional toward full realization. As more knowledge and experience are gained, professional identity may change.

Various factors, both external and internal, combine to become a part of professional development and make it a dynamic process. External factors are a major influence on a person from birth to death and include the values and beliefs of peers, parents, and significant others. These values and views have influenced and reinforced the student's concept of health care and nursing. For instance, touch as a means of communication is not acceptable in some families. Within the nursing profession, touch is an essential means of communication and care delivery that promotes individual health. Therefore, a student from a background where touch was avoided may have an aversion to its use in nursing care.

The internal factors are personal feelings and values and are shaped in great part by external factors. These internal factors are part of an individual's identity and may never change. For example, a person may enter nursing because of compassion and the desire to help others. These may be desired values that enhance nursing practice. On the other hand, a student may be uncomfortable at the thought of caring for a dying person or persons with problems related to elimination, sexuality, or disfigurement, such as clients with colostomies, AIDS, or amputations. Uneasiness or fear in these areas may affect the nursing care provided.

Throughout the educational process, students helped to recognize and manage the external and internal factors and their effects on health care delivery. Faculty members and nurses in the clinical facilities serve as models in the student's role development and socialization. These individuals may have views that are similar to those of the student. Faculty and practicing nurses may reinforce these views, or they may challenge the student's views by presenting ideas different from those held by the student. Differing views may present conflict within the student that may be stressful, but this conflict is necessary to change and imperative to the socialization process. The discussion of these feelings with role models and peers facilitates role development. Student organizations contribute to socialization and role development. Two organizations that effect professional development are the National Student Nurses' Association (NSNA) and Sigma Theta Tau (STT). The NSNA purposes include: "(a) to assume responsibility for contributing to nursing education in order to provide for the highest quality health care, (b) to provide programs representative of fundamental and current professional interests and concerns, and (c) to aid in the development of the whole person, his/her professional role, and his/her responsibility for the health care of people in all walks of life" (National Student Nurses' Association, 1986, p. 11). This organization has state as well as local constituency groups. STT inducts undergraduate and graduate students into its organization, thus contributing to the socialization process. The purposes of STT have been previously discussed. Other organizations focus on personal growth or broadening students' awareness of health care in various cultures. For instance, LasAmigas is an organization in which students volunteer health services for the poor of needy countries.

NURSING AND POLITICS

It would be remiss not to discuss nursing as it interfaces with the political system and the role of nursing in the political arena. This is an area that continues to be of importance to the professionalization process. Politics pervades the entire health care delivery system, and nursing is no exception. Nurses are involved in politics at the government level as well as within the workplace, professional nursing organizations, and the community. *Nursing: A Social Policy Statement* (ANA, 1980, p. 3) outlines:

Leadership responsibilities in five areas frequently addressed as political are: 1. the organization, delivery, and financing of health care; 2. the development of health resources; 3. preventive and environmental measures to provide for public health; 4. the development of new knowledge and technology through research; and 5. health care planning.

Even with these broad political areas identified by the ANA, before the 1970s nurses were not politically organized and, therefore, had very little influence on health care legislation. The development of formalized political action in nursing and the formation of the Nurses' Coalition for Action in Politics (N-CAP) was summarized by Rothberg (1985). In 1974, N-CAP was established as the political arm of ANA. This organization was a direct development of the work of a group of nurses from New York State who met in the early 1970s to discuss that nursing had very little structure to make an impact on major health care legislation. Impetus for this meeting came from the sense of powerlessness experienced by nurses, even though they comprise the largest group of health care providers. The group of New York nurses eventually formed the Nurses for Political Action (NPA). This organization was separate from the American Nurses Association, and its mission was "to influence health care legislation and to educate other officials and the general public on the role nurses do and can plan in the delivery of health care" (Nurses for Political Action, 1972).

Unlike the legislative focus of the ANA, the focus of the NPA was political in nature. Both groups were interested in pursuing strategies to a mutual organization of their efforts. Representatives from NPA and ANA formed a task force for this purpose. In 1973, the ANA Board of Directors voted to create a political action committee, which was known as N-CAP and is currently reorganized as **ANA-PAC (American Nurses Association-Political Action Committee).** This organization has its own board of directors and, because of tax and campaign laws, remains a separate organization from the ANA.

Many states have political action committees (PACs) to educate nurses about political activities, encourage their involvement in politics, and to raise money to support political candidates who support nursing and health care (Archer & Goehner, 1982).

Bullough & Bullough (1984) state that nurses can take action in any number of issues that need legislative action. Nurses need to review the political implications and plan their actions accordingly. When nurses are organized and work together, many issues can be brought to the public's attention and eventually be resolved. It is not uncommon today for nurses empowered by ANA to voice concerns related to health at various congressional hearings.

To be more politically active, ANA moved to Washington, D.C. in 1992. Updating nurses on legislative issues regarding health care and nursing issues is essential. This is accomplished through a variety of newsletters sent to state nursing associations, state boards, and individual nurses. One example is the monthly newsletter *Capital Update*, which informs readers about current legislative issues.

Activities, such as writing letters or attending meetings, are basic mechanisms to express an opinion or viewpoint. There have been instances where nurses have voiced opinions that resulted in policy changes for advertisements. In a wine and flower commercial, nursing was not portrayed in a professional manner. After input from nurses by way of letter, telephone calls, and telegrams, the companies changed their advertisements. A similar situation occurred with a television show depicting nurses in a traditional and nonprofessional perspective. This show was removed from the air.

It is essential for nurses to be aware of and involved in political and legislative issues. Since nurses are one of the largest groups of health care providers, they have the potential power to influence health care changes and decision making at this level.

SUMMARY

Nursing has progressed in the process of professionalization and attainment of professional status. With expanding nursing knowledge and theory development, nursing is moving closer to meeting the criteria of a profession. As in any profession, the nursing student is involved in a socialization process, which includes learning the knowledge, skills, values, and attitudes of nursing. Students are socialized into the profession through a process that includes experience in a formal educational setting where the knowledge base is learned and in guided clinical experience (practice) in a variety of health care settings. Inherent in the process is exposure to the culture of the profession for the purpose of internalization. While progressing through the nursing program, the nursing student develops in the role of a nurse. This process may be slow and difficult, or it may be a smooth, progressive change with little conscious effort. Students enter nursing with a basic idea of what it means to be a nurse. These ideas have developed from the student's interpretation of experiences with health care professionals, peers, family, the media, and others. These ideas may include both realistic and unrealistic expectations of nursing. Finally, political aspects of the profession are mentioned briefly.

▶ Questions for Discussion

1. Using the six characteristics of a profession, discuss nursing's involvement with each.
2. Do you think nursing is viewed as a profession by society and the health care system?
3. What function do specialized nursing organizations serve in terms of professional development?
4. Who has been the most influential person in developing your idea of a nurse?
5. How would you explain the socialization process?
6. What are the advantages of formalized political action in nursing?
7. What role can professional nurses play in ANA-PAC?

REFERENCES

American Nurses Association. *Bylaws.* New York: ANA; 1970.

American Nurses Association. Educational Preparation for Nurse Practitioners and Assistants to Nurses: A position paper. (Publication #G-83). Kansas City, MO: ANA; 1965.

American Nurses Association. *Nursing: A Social Policy Statement.* Kansas City, MO; 1980.

Archer, SE, & Goehner, P. *Nurses: A Political Force.* Boston: Jones & Bartlett; 1982.

Brim O, Wheeler S. *Socialization After Childhood: Two Essays.* New York: Wiley; 1966.

Brown EL. *Nursing for the Future.* New York: Russell Sage Foundation; 1948.

Bullough V, Bullough B. *History, Trends and Politics of Nursing.* Norwalk, CT: Appleton-Century-Crofts; 1984.

Cohen H. *The Nurses Quest for a Personal Identity.* Menlo Park: Addison-Wesley; 1981.

Conley M. Management effectiveness and the role making process. *J Nurs Admin.* 1974; 4:6.

Ellis JR, Hartley C. *Nursing in Today's World: Challenges, Issues and Trends.* 5th ed. Philadelphia: Lippincott; 1995.

Flexner A. Is social work a profession? *Proc Nat Conf Char.* 1915; 578–581.

Guinee K. *The Professional Nurse: Orientation, Roles and Responsibilities.* Toronto: Macmillan; 1970.

Holt J. Updating Cherry Ames. *Am J Nurs.* 1977; 77:1581–1583.

Jacox A. Professional socialization of nurses. *J NYS Nurses' Assoc.* 1973; 4:4.

Kalisch P, Kalisch B. The image of the nurse in motion pictures. *Am J Nurs.* 1982a; 82:605–611.

Kalisch P, Kalisch B. The image of nurses in novels. *Am J Nurs.* 1982:82b; 1200–1224.

Kalisch P, Kalisch B. Nurses on prime time television. *Am J Nurs.* 1982c; 82:264–270.

National Student Nurses' Association. *Getting the Pieces to Fit 86/87. A Handbook for State Associations and School Chapters.* New York: NSNA; 1986.

Nurses for Political Action. Nurses organize national action group. *News release:* July 27, 1972.

Rothberg J. The growth of political action in nursing. *Nurs Out* 1985; 33:133–135.

BIBLIOGRAPHY

Adler P. The transitional experience: An alternative view of culture shock. *J Hum Psych.* 1975; 15:4.

American Nurses Association. First position on education for nursing. *Am J Nurs.* 1965; 12:106–111.

Andreoli GK, Musser LA. Trends that may affect nursing's future. *Nurs Health Care.* 1985; 6:1.

Archer SE. Political involvement by nurses. *Recent Adv Nurs* 1987; 18:25–45.

Ashley J. Nursing and early feminism. *Am J Nurs.* 1973; 9:1465.

Bartkowski J, Swandley J. Charting nursing's course through megatrends. *Nurs Health Care.* 1985; 6:375–377.

Committee for the Study of Nursing Education. *Nursing and Nursing Education.* New York: Macmillan; 1923.

Fagin C. Can we bring order out of the chaos of nursing education? *Am J Nurs.* 1976, 1:98–105.

Hipps O. The integrated curriculum. *Am J Nurs.* 1981; 81:976–980.

Jones SL. Socialization vs. selection factors as sources of student's definition of the nurse role. *J Nurs Stud.* 1976; 13:135–138.

Kohnke M. The nurse as advocate. *Am J Nurs.* 1980; 11:2038–2040.

Passos J. Accountability: The long road back to professional practice. *J NYS Nurses' Assoc.* 1976; 7:27–28.

Schorr T. Yes, Virginia, nursing is a profession. *Am J Nurs.* 1981; 81:959.

Thompson J, Diers D. DRGs and nursing. *Health Care.* 1985; 6:435–439.

5
CHAPTER

The Health Care Delivery System

▶ **Objectives**

After studying this chapter, the student will be able to:

1. Describe the health care delivery system.
2. Describe means of classifying the formal health care delivery system.
3. Identify at least six health care providers.
4. Explain the types of health care services in the United States.
5. Discuss the various types of hospitals.
6. List several legislative and financial programs for health care.
7. Discuss factors contributing to the high cost of health care.

▶ **Questions to think about before reading the chapter**

- What are the health care agencies with which you are familiar?
- Who are the health care team members with whom you have had contact? What are their roles in the health care delivery system?
- What are some societal influences in the health care delivery system?
- What are the differences and similarities between types of hospitals?

▶ **Terms to know**

Acute care

Agency for Health Care Policy and Research (AHCPR)

Ambulatory care

Birthing center

Capitation

Center for Disease Control and Prevention (CDC)

Clinic

Community mental health center

Dentist

Diagnosis-related group (DRG)

Dietitian

Gatekeeper	Preferred provider organization (PPO)
Health care administrator	Prenatal care
Health care delivery system (HCDS)	Primary care
Health maintenance organization (HMO)	Primary prevention
Health promotion	Primary health care
Health screening	Proprietary agency
Hospice	Rehabilitation
Hospital	Respiratory therapist
Informal health care	Secondary health care
Integrated delivery system (IDS)	Secondary prevention
Joint Commission on Accreditation of Health Care Organizations (JCAHCO)	Self-care
	Skilled nursing facility (SNF)
Managed care	Social worker
Medicaid	Tertiary health care
Medicare	Tertiary prevention
National Institutes of Health (NIH)	Third-party payer
Nursing center	Universal coverage
Occupational therapist	Unlicensed assistive personnel (UAP)
Official agencies	U.S. Department of Health and Human Services (USDHHS)
Pastoral care	
Pharmacist	U.S. Public Health Service (USPHS)
Physical therapist	Voluntary agencies
Physician	Well-child center

► *Introduction*

*The **health care delivery system (HCDS)** is one of the largest industries in the United States employing over 11 million people or approximately 10% of the total work force (US Dept of Labor, 1993). The share of the gross national product (GNP) that the United States spent on health care in 1993 was 13.9 percent or a cost of over 884 billion dollars per year (Leirt, et al, 1994). It is estimated that this figure could be as high as 20 percent by 2004 if little is done to decrease the cost. These are costly figures when compared to a 6 percent GNP in 1965. The cost of health care has risen on the average 11.7 percent each year since 1965, far ex-*

ceeding any other advanced country (Knickman, 1995). Part of the reason for the increased costs has been the focus on diagnosing and treating disease and not on the promotion and protection of health. Most health insurance has paid the full cost of health care plus the encumbering high cost of technology. There has been little financial incentive for health promotion.

The HCDS may be viewed from a systems perspective as previously discussed in Chapter 2. Levey and Loomba (1973) have defined the health care system as the "totality of resources a population or society distributes in the organization and delivery of health services." They further define health services as "personal and public services performed by individuals or institutions for the purpose of maintaining or restoring health" (p. 4). Pender (1996) defines an additional aspect of health services as **health promotion,** *which refers to maintaining and enhancing well-being.*

The organization of health care delivery may be conceptualized as an open system developed around the health care needs of society. Its subsystems are the consumers and clients, professionals and paraprofessionals, and various health agencies. The suprasystem is society with its influences, such as trends in technology, cost, accessibility, political involvement, disease types and distribution, and demographics and population distribution. The entire system is influenced by the economic and sociopolitical climate of the country.

The parts of the system interact with one another in various degrees, and all respond to changes in individuals, environment, and health. The interaction of the subsystems and suprasystems aims at provision of health. The HCDS is the formal means by which Americans receive health care. Informal means for obtaining health care through cultural folk practices and personal or family resources. Figure 5–1 illustrates this formal HCDS.

THE HEALTH CARE DELIVERY SYSTEM

The HCDS in the United States is undergoing change. These changes stem from the rapidly escalating cost of health care. As mentioned earlier, in 1993 almost 14 percent of the GNP was spent on health care and without measures to curb the rapid rise, by 2004 the cost of health care is estimated to be 20 percent of the GNP. Many factors have contributed to this problem. Historically consumers and providers of health care had little incentive to control the amount of care provided or the related costs of care. **Third-party payers,** not the consumer of the health care, paid the cost. An oversupply of specialists has also contributed to the rapid rise in health care cost.

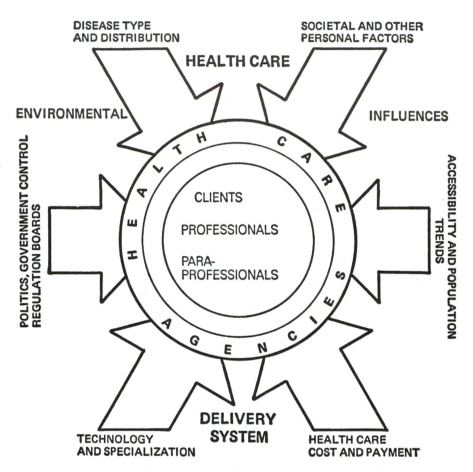

Figure 5–1. The health care delivery system.

Consumers also had little interest in controlling costs because they frequently had little contact with actually paying for the cost of health care. Employer- or government-paid insurance for health care contributed to overconsumption of health care benefits. Consumers felt they were entitled to the "best" health care, but there were few controls on unnecessary treatment or surgery. For example the use of computerized axial tomographic (CAT) scans have risen 400 percent in the last 10 years. The more expensive health care became, the more insurance or protection consumers wanted. The more insurance consumers had, the more physicians and hospitals used expensive technology. More recently, consumers have been faced with higher premiums for health care, higher deductibles, and have had to bear more of the cost of health care. Health care providers have also been faced with excessive litigation, causing many physicians to practice "defensive" medicine by ordering unnecessary tests, thus driving up the cost of health care.

The recent shift in health care has been to more competition. The power in the health care system has shifted from those who provide care to those to pay for it. Currently, the traditional acute-care facilities, hospitals, have been faced with a drop in the number of patients as patients are discharged earlier and fewer patients are admitted to hospitals. This has shifted the need for health care from the hospital setting to areas outside the hospital, in the community.

The formal HCDS is a complex social organization. Unlike that of other countries, the health care system in the United States does not have a person in charge of administering the system. It is an interdependent system whose purpose is health care of persons, families, and groups. Health care providers in the system are professionals and paraprofessional with special preparation in addressing health care needs. Two classification methods are presented here to describe the formal structure of the HCDS. Comprehending the terminology can help to better understand the components of the system.

Classification of Health Care Delivery

The first method of classifying the HCDS is as official (established by law) or public, voluntary or nonprofit, and profit-making agencies. All three types of agencies are concerned with prevention of illness and promotion and maintenance of health.

The **official agencies** or public health agencies are supported primarily through the government, with funds from taxes, and are broad in scope. The official agencies' main functions are to "administer and coordinate programs, conduct research, analyze statistics and set standards and qualifications" (Stewart, 1979, p. 25). One example of an official agency is the **United States Public Health Service (USPHS).** The USPHS is obligated to prevent communicable disease and promote the community's health (**Centers for Disease Control and Prevention—CDC**). Agencies are established at the local, state, and national levels, with each lower level having specific responsibilities and functions coordinated at the national level. For example, at the local level, the health department usually has the responsibility of identifying environmental and personal health care needs of a particular geographic area and organizing sources and efforts to meet these needs. The span of interest broadens at the state and national levels.

Another federal government agency is the **Agency for Health Care Policy and Research (AHCPR),** which was established in 1989 to "enhance the quality, appropriateness, and effectiveness of health care services and access to these services" (**U.S. Department of Health and Human Services,** 1994). This agency conducts and sponsors health services research and develops and suggests practice guidelines for health care problems. Current examples of some of these guidelines include acute pain management and management of cancer pain, urinary incontinence, pressure ulcers, and sickle cell anemia. Each of these complete guidelines are available to health care practitioners and educators, and a patient guide is also available for consumers by calling 1–800–358–9295 or by writing to the AHCPR Publications Clearinghouse, P.O. Box 8547, Silver Spring, MD, 20907.

The National Institute for Nursing Research (NINR) is another public agency that is part of the **National Institutes of Health (NIH).** The purpose of NINR is to award research grants related to patient care, health promotion, and disease prevention.

The second type of HCDS organization is the **voluntary agencies** or private nonprofit groups that are supported by donations and gifts, third-party payment, and personal payment and respond to a specific need of the community. This type of organization is not profit making, and it has no official status or governmental funding. Funds for these groups come from a variety of sources, such as contributions, fees for service, fund raising, dues, investments, gifts, publications, and grants (Turner, 1977, p. 480).

The nonprofit or voluntary type of agency may have subdivisions at the local, regional, or national levels and is organized to enhance the total health care delivery effort. These agencies are autonomous and usually have a board of directors who determine the leadership of the organization, set its policies, and conduct the affairs of the organization. Membership on the board is composed primarily of nonprofessional volunteers. Volunteer agencies can be divided into four groups: (1) those that rely on contributions and donations, such as the American Heart Association or the American Cancer Society; (2) those that are private foundations accountable to a board, such as the W.K. Kellogg Foundation; (3) the professional organizations such as the American Nurses Association, who provide service to members and establish standards for practice and research; and (4) coordinating agencies such as the United Fund (Lancaster & Lancaster, 1984).

The last major type is the **proprietary agency** or privately owned agency. Some types of facilities that are part of this organizational framework are some hospitals, diagnostic centers, private home health care, skilled care facilities, and private practitioners' services. Some nurses, physicians, dentists, psychologists, and social workers are private practitioners.

The major focus of the HCDS has been on illness and disease processes. However, health care delivery has shifted from the treatment of illness to *prevention* of illness and promotion and maintenance of health. Along with this move toward health promotion, Yeaworth (1983) states that people are now expected to assume responsibility for their own health, not just illness care. As people reduce known risk factors associated with different illnesses, their health status can improve.

Several factors may be responsible for the shift in emphasis on prevention and treatment of illness to emphasis on health promotion and maintenance. Historically, health care and the work of the physician have been aimed at illness treatment or cure. The ability to control or eliminate most communicable diseases has contributed to the shift in focus. Since the late 1800s, there has been a dramatic shift in health priorities. Many of the communicable diseases that existed at the turn of the century have now been controlled through vaccines and immunizations. Some examples include poliomyelitis, smallpox, German measles, and other childhood diseases. This has led to a shift in the incidence of chronic diseases, and thus the move in health priorities from a cure orientation to health promotion and disease prevention (McMahon & Berlin, 1981).

Another factor is a change in the individual's perception of illness. Today, people are more aware of health and health-promoting behaviors and often view health care as a right rather than a privilege. As the illness needs of society are addressed, the need for health promotion and illness prevention is more apparent. Finally, viewing the person holistically, which encompasses looking at the person and environmental influences, contributes to the shift in health care orientation.

A second method of classifying the HCDS is through levels of prevention, as described by Leavell and Clark (1965). In their writings, levels of prevention are described as **primary prevention,** or the prevention of disease by measures to promote optimum health; **secondary prevention,** the early diagnosis and treatment of a disease; and **tertiary prevention,** rehabilitation of the person following a disability.

Although many textbooks and references use the levels of prevention as an organizing modality, these terms are defined differently. Some of this confusion arises from the use of the terms *primary, secondary,* and *tertiary health care.* These terms describe different levels of care for a person entering the HCDS with an actual or suspected illness. The use of these terms is very different from the levels of prevention. Primary care is the person's first contact with the HCDS, or entry into the system; secondary care is cure and restoration, and tertiary care is specialized and sophisticated care of a person with an illness that occurs infrequently and for which high levels of skill and technology are needed.

Shamansky and Clausen (1980) suggest using a more widely understood terminology for the levels based on the classic levels described by Leavell and Clark: (1) prevention, (2) early diagnosis and treatment, (3) rehabilitation.

Prevention

Prevention care or health and wellness promotion prevents or delays the occurrence of illness and promotes healthy lifestyles. Some examples of preventive health care programs include immunizations and vaccines for polio, smallpox, and typhoid; better sanitation; and health education in areas such as nutrition, risk factors, benefits of exercise, stress management, and prenatal classes. Safety programs in industry, recreation departments, and sanitation facilities are also part of prevention.

Prevention services are provided in nonspecific societal settings as well as specific facilities. For example, health education may be provided in a school or through an organization such as the American Heart Association. More specific settings are **HMOs (Health Maintenance Organizations)** and **birthing centers.**

Early Diagnosis

Early diagnosis and treatment of illness, the second level of prevention, is in the presymptomatic or early phase of illness and the client's response to illness. The largest segment of the formal HCDS is aimed at this level of prevention. This level includes **health screening** and **acute care.** Screening is done to detect an illness at an early stage. Examples of screenings at this level include breast self-examination, early detection and treatment of high blood pressure, early detection of cervical cancer with the Pap test, detection of phenylketonuria (PKU) in infants, hearing tests, the Denver Developmental Screening Test for growth and development delays, and VDRL for sexually transmitted diseases.

This level also includes acute care, which is often the most expensive type of care, since it usually requires admission to an acute short-term care facility such as a hospital. These facilities provide concentrated and intense services over a short time period. Many Americans seek health care only after a problem has been identified or the symptoms are too acute for **self-care.** Early diagnosis and treatment services are provided primarily in specific settings such as hospitals, physicians' offices, outpatient clinics, short-term community treatment centers, and community mental health centers.

Rehabilitation

The third level of prevention, rehabilitation, has gained emphasis because the life expectancy of Americans is increasing. With longevity, there is an increase in the incidence of chronic, long-term illnesses. Many persons with chronic illnesses are seen in ambulatory clinics for continued monitoring and treatment. Some of these include hypertension, cardiovascular rehabilitation, and diabetic clinics, as well as renal dialysis centers.

Rehabilitation involves assessing strengths and weaknesses of the client; facilitating development of client strengths and assisting in coping with limitations; and teaching self-care measures following an acute illness. The family and clients are also assisted through stages of death and grieving as necessary. Rehabilitation facilities are needed as a transitional phase for persons with mental or physical ailments that require a period of supervision to help them return to their optimal level of functioning. Facilities at this level include rehabilitation centers, halfway houses, specialty hospitals, clinics, long-term facilities, nursing homes, skilled care facilities, home health agencies, and specialty groups (e.g., Alcoholics Anonymous, Reach to Recovery, and ostomy clubs). **Hospices** address the health of terminally ill clients and their families. Hospices are discussed in more detail later in this chapter and in Chapter 6. In keeping with the systems approach, increased societal value, in terms of health and health care—can be said to be placed not only on the subsystem of client but also on the subsystems of family and community and the suprasystem of the larger society.

Factors Influencing the Health Care Delivery System

In discussion of the various classification methods that make up the HCDS, the complexity of the system becomes evident. The complexity is compounded by numerous societal influences within and without the system:

- Trends in technology
- Rising cost of health care
- Emphasis on illness and cure rather than health promotion
- Inadequate coordination of services
- Disproportional accessibility to health care
- Number of people without insurance or underinsured
- Varied types of health care personnel
- Political involvements
- Disease type and distribution
- Other personal factors

Recent rapid advances in technology, increases in automation, and use of computers have led to the use of specialized and more complex equipment, requiring increased expense. In many instances, agencies have had to expand and renovate existing facilities to accommodate the new equipment. Additional personnel have been necessary to operate and maintain equipment. Health area employment from 1975 to 1990 grew at a faster rate than the rate of employment in the United States (Salsberg & Kovner, 1995). Costs have skyrocketed as a result. In some instances, when new technology has been introduced, entire departments have developed. For example, formerly all types of critically ill patients might have been found in one intensive or critical care unit. Today these patients are placed in specialty critical care units such as surgical intensive care, medical intensive care, or coronary intensive care units.

In spite of the increased technology, there are still persons who do not have complete access to the HCDS as a result of geographical constraints and cost factors. While most major health centers are located in urban areas where there is a greater concentration of consumers, a variety of factors related to a lack of financial and other resources contribute to inadequate access of the poor and uninsured to quality health care. Also, consumers in rural areas may have limited access to health care facilities and may have difficulty getting to the major centers for specialized care and equipment. Some examples of rural limitation in health care delivery are Appalachia rural migrant work areas, and remote Indian reservations.

The changing work force in health care delivery has had some dramatic effects. The recent shift to a competition-based system that relies on market forces has created new employment opportunities for nurses and health personnel. Positions for professional nurses in acute-care facilities have become more limited in the past few years as a result of changes in these settings. In response to an oversupply of acute-care beds, hospitals have closed or combined units and have downsized their entire operation in response to declining hospital admissions and increasing costs, resulting in fewer professional nursing positions and an increased use of **unlicensed assistive personnel (UAP).** These "nurse extenders" are recruited and trained "on the job" as support personnel to the professional staff. While these positions are helpful to streamline operations in nonpatient settings, such as housekeeping and food service, they do not have the knowledge to be placed in patient care situations where judgment and critical thinking are essential.

Although there appears to be an oversupply of registered nurses and a limited number of employment opportunities for nurses in acute-care settings, a long-term shortage of professional nurses is projected for the year 2005 (PEW, 1991). Aiken (1995) describes a shortage of nurses educated at the baccalaureate level, those who should be responsible for complex patient care problems in acute-care settings and the community. One reason for the shortage is that students take longer to graduate; only 53 percent of full-time students graduated within 6 years. The supply of qualified faculty to meet the demands of increased enrollments is also limited. The average age of the registered nurse population is also changing. In 1992 it was 43 years (Erwin, 1993).

Nurses are in an ideal position to move from the treatment-oriented and expensive mode of illness care to health protection and promotion in community settings. One way nurses are making an impact is through the use of nurse-managed centers or **nursing centers.** This is not a new concept but one that has enjoyed a resurgence of interest. Primary care is the type of care rendered at these clinics (Holthaus, 1993).

Government control and legislation also have an impact on health care. Efforts are constantly being made by medical and political groups to change or influence the delivery of health care services in order to improve care for more people. One of these efforts was the 1965 passage of the two much publicized amendments to the Social Security Act, Title XVIII **(Medicare)** and Title XIX **(Medicaid).** Medicare provides a federally administered program of health insurance for the aged. This includes hospitalization insurance financed through social security taxes and a voluntary program of supplementary benefits financed by matching contributions. Medicaid provides a program of grants to be distributed to needy persons of any age for medical assistance. In 1993 both of these programs spent $272.1 billion for health care, which was 30.8 percent of health spending in the United States and 70.2 percent of all health care finances by public funding (Levit, et al., 1994).

In 1983 the federal government used a prospective payment system for Medicare using **diagnosis-related groups (DRGs)** to determine and control health care costs. Over time DRGs have decreased hospital stays because reimbursement is now predetermined. Hospitals lose money if the hospital stay is longer than the reimbursement, and likewise, they can save money if the hospital stay is shorter.

Reimbursement for health care and the staggering number of people who are underinsured or lack insurance have created a financial burden. In 1992, 17.4 percent of the nonelderly population were uninsured (Levit, et al., 1994). Private health insurance paid about 30 percent of all health expenditures in 1993. Managed health care organizations provide a means for health care to be planned to effectively control costs. Consumers who belong to a **managed care** system select a **primary care** provider (e.g., family practitioner, pediatrician, nurse practitioner) under the managed system. This primary provider is the **gatekeeper** and makes the decisions on referrals to other specialists. Many insurance companies have been moving into managed care as a way to manage increased costs of health care. Health maintenance organizations (HMOs) and **preferred provider organizations (PPOs)** are examples of managed care organizations.

Hospitals faced with an oversupply of beds from low occupancy and increased operating and maintenance costs are merging with other institutions to create **integrated delivery systems (IDS).** These alliances pull together the entire continuum of care under one system, with the focus of care on primary care to provide more cost-effective care. A fully operational system uses hospitals, clinics, physicians, nurses, subacute care, facilities, home health care, pharmacy, and durable medical goods and covers a broad geographic area (Stahl, 1995).

Health care reform is slow. Although several proposals have been introduced in Congress to help deal with the rising costs of health care, no consensus has been reached. Some of the proposals favor strict government control while others support private industry. Issues to be discussed include the type of coverage and who should be covered. **Universal coverage** would provide coverage for everyone without exclusion for prior conditions. Another question is whether funding should come from taxes or from other sources. Whether payment is to be direct or by a third party is a major concern for nurses, pharmacists, psychologists, social workers, and other health care providers. Without reimbursement, these professionals would have decreased control over health care costs. This could result in a decrease in client care quality, since the major control of care would not rest with the entire health care team.

Disease types and distribution have had an influence on the HCDS. For example, until the mid 1960s, tuberculosis hospitals were common, but with current preventive and treatment measures to control the disease, tuberculosis hospitals are no longer necessary. Areas that have a high incidence of particular types of disease may require different health care facilities from other areas. Within highly populated urban areas, there may be an increased incidence of certain types of disease not found in rural areas. Therefore, the health care facilities may differ according to the health needs of the population. For example, for some populations living in older housing developments, teaching and preventive services concerning lead content of paint and possible lead poisoning are necessary.

In light of the definitions of person, health, and environment, it becomes evident that many factors influence one's perception and definition of health. These factors include genetic and environmental influences, cultural responses, prenatal care issues, personal beliefs, number of people living at or below the poverty level, accidents, values, and life experiences. For example, in American society, the well-being of individuals is believed to be a generally accepted right regardless of the individual's color, sex, age, economic or social status, or creed. Through the HCDS, society has sought methods for realization of this belief. While well-being as a right for all is a belief of many Americans, it has not been formulated in legal terms.

Another influence on the HCDS is the increased life expectancy of consumers. More geriatric clients present unique health care problems and concerns, including management of long-term illness.

HEALTH CARE SERVICES

Individuals can enter the HCDS at any one of various levels, which is characteristic of an open system. Once in the HCDS, the individual may obtain services for prevention, identification, and treatment of health problems or rehabilitation. Although some agencies may address all three areas of health care, they usually focus on one. For example, the major focus of hospitals has been and continues to be acute care. As a result of cost-containment efforts and increased emphasis on health promotion, hospitals have experienced a decrease in census. This has necessitated increased efforts toward alternative use of the hospital facilities for health promotion and rehabilitation programs. For the same reasons, outpatient medical and surgical services have also expanded. The following section considers the agencies and referral systems that address preventive health care of individuals or groups, diagnosis and treatment, and rehabilitation health care. Within each level some services overlap.

Services for Health Promotion

American society relies on the individual to assume responsibility for health care. In the U.S. Public Health Service publication *Healthy People 2000, National Health Promotion and Disease Preventions Objectives* (1990) three major goals for the nation are identified: to increase the span of healthy life for Americans, reduce health disparities among Americans, and achieve access to preventive services for all Americans. The document is organized into 22 priority areas within three categories: health promotion, health protection, and illness prevention. Health-promoting behaviors can focus on physical activity and fitness; improved nutritional intake; less tobacco, alcohol, and other drug use; improved mental health; less violent and abusive behavior, and enhanced educational programs. Health-protecting behaviors can reduce unintentional injuries and improve occupational safety, environmental health, and oral health. Preventive services are directed to improve maternal and infant health; increase immunizations; reduce the incidence of heart disease, stroke, sexually transmitted diseases, cancer, diabetes, and other disabling conditions; and prevent and control HIV infection. These services for health promotion are also consistent with protocols for delivery of health care discussed in *Nursing's Agenda for Health Care Reform* (National League for Nursing, 1991).

To promote health, the client is given information and other resources; however, it is the individual's responsibility to carry out the health-promoting behaviors and to follow through with health promotion practices. Because health promotion services are also provided in numerous nontraditional settings (e.g., churches, schools, homes), they are referred to as health promotion structures.

Prenatal Center

A **prenatal care** center, one type of health-promoting center, may be established in a local community facility such as a church or school or individual's home, and care is usually provided by community health agencies. Health care services focus on the changing family's feelings, attitudes, and expectations. For instance, an expectant family may receive education concerning growth and development of the child to be born, financial planning, nutritional requirements, physical changes of the mother, birthing, child care, and psychosocial responses to a new family member. In addition, support may be provided to families for problems resulting from changes in the family because of the expected infant.

Birthing Centers

Birthing centers or childbearing centers provide a homelike setting with the presence of family members and significant others during the delivery of a child. They thus allow maintenance of the family unit during a significant and critical life moment. Professional staff members, usually including a midwife, are readily available. A birthing center may adjoin a hospital or be an independent community facility.

Well-Child Centers

Well-child centers are established to assist the family in the care of their growing child. Centers may be located in established clinics, schools, or churches. These centers provide for health assessment (physical examination, developmental screening procedures), illness prevention (immunizations, parenting education, home safety practices), and nutritional counseling.

Educational Systems

Elementary and secondary educational systems have incorporated preventive health teaching into their curriculums. Children and adolescents participate in courses where concepts aimed at health maintenance and self-care are discussed. A recent focus in curriculums has been on healthy lifestyles, human sexuality, and chemical abuse. Students are taught basic skills in first aid, cardiopulmonary resuscitation (CPR), and the Heimlich maneuver. Screening programs are conducted within schools for early detection of hearing, visual, and dental problems, along with growth and developmental obstacles such as obesity and scoliosis. Disease is prevented through immunization programs, and support is given to students for individual concerns through guidance and counseling services.

Health Maintenance Organizaztions

HMOs provide health care services. The HMO arrangement is designed to prevent illness and decrease the need for hospitalization or the length of hospitalization. They are financed by a prepaid fee for services (capitation). The client periodically pays an established sum in return for preventive services and educational materials, as well as comprehensive health care services. Cornett (1984) describes some of the general characteristics of an HMO which are still used today and are the basis for managed care programs. These include: (1) voluntary enrollment; (2) fixed, prepaid premium; and (3) health care services provided by staff with outside referrals as necessary.

There are four basic types of HMOs.

1. *Staff.* Health care services are provided by an established group practice; professionals are employed directly by the HMO.
2. *Group.* The HMO contracts with a group practice to provide health care. The group is compensated on a capitation basis.
3. *Network.* Two or more group practices with various specialties are contracted to provide health care.
4. *Individualized Practice Associations (IPA).* Individual professionals are contracted to provide health care to prepaid clients as well as maintaining their own clients (Cornett, 1984; Deeds, 1985).

Some employers provide health care benefits to their employees under group membership in HMOs. Although the focus is on prevention, early diagnosis, and treatment, rehabilitation services are also provided. An advantage of the HMO is cost containment as an alternative means of financing health care services. Over the past 10 years HMOs have continued to grow at a rate of 4 to 5 percent with about 40 million people enrolled in 570 plans nationwide (Relman, 1994). HMOs are more prominent on the East and West coasts. For example, California has the highest percentage of enrollees (33.4 percent) followed by Massachusetts (30.9 percent) (Iglehart, 1994).

Preferred Provider Organization

Health care services in a PPO are similar to those of an HMO, but clients are able to select a specific health care provider from an approved list of providers. Unlike the HMO, there is no physical structure, and the client has more selection of provider. In a PPO, the network of health care providers agree to deliver services to enrollees at a predetermined fee in return for the PPO providing patients to them. Patients using providers outside the PPO usually pay an extra fee.

Industry

Industry has become a major setting for health promotion. Health screening programs for employees for hearing, visual, and other health-related problems (e.g., alcoholism, diabetes, and hypertension) have been established. Safety measures through industrial and governmental control, such as the federal Occupational Safety and Health Act (OSHA), have been instituted in the areas of noise abatement and environmental hazard control. Other primary health services offered are health education, counseling, and referral services for identified problems.

The changing view of Americans to include more health promotion activities in their daily routines since the 1970s has resulted in the development of wellness centers and wellness programs. No longer are infectious diseases the major cause of mortality in the United States, as they once were during the early part of this century.

The CDC (1994) estimates that 47 percent of premature deaths of Americans could be decreased by changes in behaviors, another 17 percent could be avoided by reducing environmental risks, but only 11 percent can be prevented by better access to medical treatment.

It is not unusual to find an increase in health promotion programs in business and industry. The rising cost of illness care has spurred the interest in health-promoting activities as a means to improve health and decrease the chance of illnesses developing.

Wellness centers can be multi- or unidimensional depending on the population being served. Such populations can include employees, individuals, families, or community groups. Typical services provided by wellness centers include emphasis on self-care and responsibility for health promotion; diet and nutritional counseling; exercise programs; stress management; drug and substance abuse counseling; blood pressure screening; womens' health care; smoke cessation clinics; environmental hazard awareness; and risk reduction.

Services for Early Diagnosis and Treatment

The individual may enter the health care system at this level when an illness process has been identified by the individual, family, community member, or health professional. As in prevention, the individual usually has the ultimate responsibility for seeking and accepting care. Individuals must recognize when they are ill and must assume, to a certain degree, the "sick role" as described in Chapter 2. There are a variety of health services to meet these health needs.

Hospitals

Hospitals are the major centers for early diagnosis and treatment. This is probably the most familiar health care structure. The hospital is an age-old institution with a focus shifting from custodial care to a vast interdisciplinary center for health care and research. Its main purpose is to provide health care services for acute and critical health problems. Hospitals have developed from social needs in various periods of history. Hospitals were first established by the early Christians as a penitence for receiving grace and carrying out the teachings of Christ. Many of these early hospitals were actually only roadside shelters, vastly different from the highly complex, bureaucratic systems of today.

The great advances in science and technology in the care of the sick and injured enhanced the development of hospitals. As schools of medicine improved after the turn of the 20th century, so did hospitals, since these were the facilities in which physicians care for their patients. Over the years, hospitals have changed from charitable institutions to specialized centers that serve the community's health care needs. The terms *medical center* and *health care center* have been used to describe a broadened concept of health care services within hospitals.

Hospitals are bureaucratic, highly organized, complex institutions with many departments and health care providers. Communication is carried on via an intricate, structured social network. Typical departments within the hospital include administration, nursing, medicine, dietary, pharmacy, pastoral care, laboratory, social services, and occupational, speech, and physical therapy.

As major centers for care of the ill and injured, hospitals today are categorized in various classifications. One classification is based on whether they offer short- or long-term care. Hospitals also may be differentiated by their primary means of financial support, either public or private. Private hospitals may be associated with nonprofit groups such as religious denominations and other private associations, or with profit-making groups. Public hospitals include federal, state, county, and city facilities. Hospitals are also classified according to size, ranging anywhere from 20 beds in a small rural community to over 1000 beds in an urban or university setting.

Arrangement of hospitals by generalization or specialization is another type of classification. A general hospital is an example of a nonspecialty hospital. Persons of all ages and health care needs are admitted to such an institution. Usually general hospitals comprise patient care units such as medical, surgical, urological, oncological, orthopedic, and psychiatric. One type of hospital established for specialized care is the mental health facility, which is equipped to deal with alterations in a person's psychosocial health. Other examples of specialized hospitals are children's hospitals, which concern themselves with childhood diseases. These hospitals admit children directly or by referral from another health care setting. Additional examples of specialized hospitals are those for maternity, orthopedic problems, and alcohol and drug abuse.

Most major urban areas have many general hospitals. A number of these were built after WWII under the Hill-Burton program, when the population was concentrated in the cities. With population shifts, more hospitals were built in the suburbs. This poses a current problem for the urban hospitals. While smaller community hospitals have until the recent past been filled to capacity, the larger, older urban hospitals have had many empty beds. This is due in part to the inconvenient location of many urban hospitals. Hospitals today meet needs other than direct care of the sick. These needs may include biomedical research and multidisciplinary health education.

Hospitals are licensed through the state and must meet minimum standards. In addition to licensure, hospitals may participate in voluntary accreditation through the **Joint Commission on Accreditation of Health Care Organizations (JCAHO).** This accreditation indicates the attainment of high standards with eligibility for federal funding and affiliation with education programs.

In all of these health care facilities, the major focus is on the client who already has a potential or identified illness. Health care workers in these settings may assist with preventive and rehabilitative measures; however, their main function is to treat illness.

Ambulatory Care Centers

Nurse-managed centers are community-based, nurse-run clinics. Types of services include birthing centers, wellness programs, long-term continuity care, support services for caregivers of patients with debilitating diseases such as Alzheimer's (Walker, 1994).

Ambulatory Surgery

In response to health care costs of in-hospital surgery and less government and third party regulation, ambulatory or same-day surgery centers have increased. Some are free-standing investor-owned facilities and others are affiliated with hospitals. Approximately half of all surgical procedures are now being done safely on an out-patient basis (Relman, 1994).

Clinics

Another type of agency serving early diagnosis and treatment needs is the **clinic.** Clinics may be affiliated with a hospital but may be independently operated. As an **ambulatory care** facility, the clinic service is provided to clients who require short-term health care or follow-up care after hospitalization. Although clinics span all levels of health care delivery, a large proportion of them provide treatment and diagnosis of disease for ambulatory clients.

Clients enter the clinic, obtain treatment, and return home. Clinics are usually organized to meet potential and actual health care needs of specific groups of clients. Some examples are clinics for eye disorders, medical clinics for general internal disorders such as ulcers and heart disease, surgical clinics for minor surgery or follow-up after surgery in the hospital, orthopedic clinics for clients with problems such as fractures & joint replacements, dermatology clinics for skin disorders, and weight control clinics for obese clients. These clinics are staffed by physicians, nurses, and other care providers such as dietitians and social workers. "Free clinics" were quite popular during the late 1960s and early 1970s for persons unable to pay for health care services. They were usually funded by government grants. Recently many have been forced to close as a result of financial difficulty caused by the decrease in government funding.

Physicians' Offices and Private Practice

The major focus of health care delivery in physicians' offices consists of diagnosis, treatment, and follow-up care for specific illness. This care is usually given on an ambulatory basis, as only a small percentage of the clients are hospitalized. Entry for most people into the health care delivery system is through the physician. Many physicians practice medicine in established offices and have privileges at nearby hospitals for the admission of clients. Physicians are reimbursed by a fee for services, which may be covered by the client's health insurance or are reimbursed as part of a capitation or managed care program.

Community Mental Health Centers

The final setting to be discussed is the **community mental health center,** where a broad range of mental health services are provided. Since the mid-1960s, the focus of care for these clients has been in a community setting rather than the hospital, and for this reason these centers are generally organized as outpatient centers. Clients are referred for diagnosis and treatment of emotional dysfunctions or dysfunctions related to crisis. It is the aim of the clinic setting to help clients function within society while participating in treatment close to their home and families (Lancaster & Lancaster, 1984).

Services for Rehabilitation

The goal of **rehabilitation** is the facilitation of a person's optimal level of functioning. The individual is encouraged to attain maximum ability to function and to develop a realistic view of strengths and limitations. Clients usually enter rehabilitation facilities by referrals from health care providers.

The goals of agencies serving clients' rehabilitation needs are restoration to optimum lifestyle functioning or assisting persons through the dying process. Some people are able to achieve these goals, while others are limited in progress because of the extent of their illness.

Specialized Rehabilitation Hospitals

Rehabilitation hospitals provide extended care for clients who no longer require the acute care services of a general hospital but need further care and training to cope with their illness or change in functioning. Specialized equipment and personnel are available to deal with long-term problems. One type of client admitted to this facility is a person with a cerebral vascular accident (stroke). Rehabilitation includes relearning the normal activities of daily living, such as dressing, eating, walking, and talking. Another type of rehabilitation client is one with a spinal cord injury resulting in paralysis. Rehabilitation includes learning to carry on activities of daily living within the restriction of change in functioning, such as confinement to a wheelchair or limited use of extremities.

Skilled Nursing Facilities

Skilled nursing facilities (SNF) have increased in number since the Medicare and Medicaid enactment of 1965. Under this amendment, nursing homes could qualify for benefits if certain federal regulations were met. Clients no longer needing acute care in a hospital setting but still needing skilled care could be cared for in an SNF for continued treatment at a lower cost. Clients in SNFs receive this skilled care and rehabilitation service, with the goal of reaching their optimal level of functioning within the facility or in their homes.

Hospices

The hospice movement began in the United States in the late 1960s. Hospices have developed to provide many services for the terminally ill and to provide for life at a quality level for terminally ill persons, their families, and significant others. The goal of the hospice movement is to maintain persons in their home environment and improve the quality of life. *Hospice* is the concept of supportive therapy that provides short-term relief for the caregiver. It provides for management of uncontrolled pain and is an alternative to acute care (Aroskar, 1985). The hospice also provides a source of emotional support and assistance through the grieving process for the individual and significant others. Bereavement care is provided to the family following the individual's death.

Community Health Agencies

Community health agencies are established to meet health needs of individuals, families, groups, and communities. They include public health agencies, home nursing services, visiting nurse associations, and nursing clinics and centers. Community agencies may function as clinics for ambulatory clients or be structured so that the health care provider sees the client within the home setting. Since the community agencies are concerned about the health needs of a diverse clientele, the skills of various health providers are required. The community health practitioner must be skilled in assessing community needs in relation to social and health problems, and be adept at applying control measures to deal with the identified problems. Clients are referred to the agencies for learning health promotion and health maintenance activities. Type and extent of care is dependent on the health needs of the client.

In all the services discussed, there is potential for overlap among prevention, early detection and diagnosis, and rehabilitation. For convenience, the major focus of health care has determined the services' placement within each level.

HEALTH CARE PROVIDERS

Health care providers make up an interdisciplinary work force that is the infrastructure of the HCDS. There are various health care providers whose common concern is the consumer. Traditionally, health care providers have been known as the health care team, which consisted of the patient, nurse, and physician. However, the influences of the HCDS, particularly that of specialization, have caused this definition to change and broaden. With increased specialization, additional types of health care providers have developed and have interdependent and collaborative roles. Over 11 million persons or about 10 percent of the work force in the United States are employed in health care or health-care–related areas (U.S. Department of Labor, 1993). These providers are now part of the health team. The interdependence of these roles, with the client as the central focus, is illustrated in Figure 5–2.

The discussion in this chapter is limited to the following health care providers: dentist (DDS), dietitian (RD), health care administra-

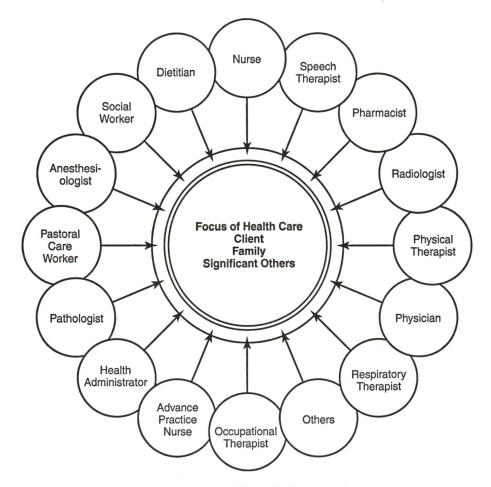

Figure 5–2. Interdependence of health care providers.

tor, occupational therapist (OT), pastoral care workers, pharmacist, physical therapist (LPT), physician (MD or DO), respiratory therapist (RT), and social worker (SW). The nurse as a member of the health team will be discussed in Chapter 6.

Dentists

Dentists provide for preventive care of the mouth and treatment of oral disorders. This includes tooth repair and extraction, filling of cavities, and making dentures. Several types of personnel may provide for dentistry needs. A dentist usually has a 4-year undergraduate degree plus 3 to 4 years of dental school. After completion of the program, licensing is mandatory through a state board examination. Dental hygienists are allied health professionals who provide care in limited aspects of dentistry (e.g., cleaning of teeth, providing fluoride treatment, and dental health care teaching).

Dietitian

The **dietitian** works to identify and meet nutritional needs of the client and supervises nutrition and food service in a variety of settings. This takes such forms as providing for selection and preparation of special diets (religious-cultural, e.g., vegetarian, kosher, or ethnic dishes; illness-related, e.g., sodium-restricted and low-cholesterol diets). The dietitian may work with individuals and groups of people in providing diet counseling and teaching. These groups may include obese, diabetic, or pregnant clients. Health diet planning may be recommended to well populations. For instance, dietitians are hired to work in school systems, businesses, and industries. Educational preparation consists of a minimum of a bachelor's degree with a major in food and nutrition. A master's degree is required for many positions. The American Dietetic Association is active in establishing criteria for dietetic curriculums as well as approving internships for further study.

Health Care Administrator

The **health care administrator's** principal function is management of a health care agency such as a hospital or community service. The educational preparation of administrators requires course work in economics and finance, short- and long-term health care planning, and program evaluation. A bachelor's degree is required, with a master's degree recommended. Many universities now offer a master's degree in hospital administration.

Occupational Therapist

Occupational therapists use purposeful activity to promote health and prevent disability. Individuals with psychosocial, developmental, and physical limitations are assisted by the occupational therapist to develop skills that promote activities of daily living and psychological, social, and economic adjustments. Educational preparation is a bachelor's degree followed by a 6- to 12-month internship. Certification is obtained through the American Occupational Therapy Association.

Pastoral Care Worker

Pastoral care provides for the spiritual needs of the individual and family members. Clergy, religious, and other persons in pastoral care provide a valuable and necessary service for spiritual counseling and support. Educational preparation is varied. Programs continue to be developed to provide education to persons in pastoral care. These programs focus on the response of individuals to health-related situations like stress, dying, illness, and crisis as they relate to religious and spiritual needs. Clinical pastoral education programs (CPE) are recommended as training for these positions.

Pharmacist

The **pharmacist** is trained in the science of drugs and their preparation. Pharmacists are responsible for preparing and dispensing prescribed medications and acting as consultants to other health team members concerning medications. In some settings, the pharmacy assistant is responsible for the distribution of medication to patients, and the pharmacist assists in monitoring and evaluating the medication's action and effect. Minimum educational preparation for a pharmacist is a 5-year collegiate program with a major in pharmacology.

Physical Therapist

The **physical therapist's** role as a health team member is working with clients who have musculoskeletal problems resulting from illness, developmental delay, or injury. The physical therapist assists these individuals to improve functional ability, reduce pain, and increase muscle strength and mobility through therapeutic measures such as heat application, manipulation, ultrasound, and massage. Educational preparation for a physical therapist is a baccalaureate degree with a major in physical therapy. Registration is through the American Registry of Physical Therapists.

Physician

Physicians are persons legally authorized to practice medicine. They are able to diagnose, prescribe, and treat disease and injury. The physician is responsible for the medical diagnosis and treatment of the client. The medical team includes the intern, resident, and staff physician. The medical student may also be a part of the team. A physician usually has a 4-year undergraduate degree followed by 3 to 4 years of medical school. Courses consist of basic sciences and clinical experience. The last 2 years of medical school usually consist of clerkship in local hospitals where patient contact begins. A doctor of medicine degree (MD) is awarded at the completion of medical school. Education after graduation is usually a 2-to-4-year residency in a specialty area. Doctors of osteopathy (DO) follow the same type

TABLE 5–1. SUMMARY OF HEALTH CARE PROVIDERS

Provider	Recommended Education	Focus
Dentist	• Baccalaureate degree • 3–4 yr dental school, licensure required	• Health care of mouth • Treatment of oral disorders (dentures, fillings, extractions, etc.)
Dietitian	• Baccalaureate degree • Optional internships	• Diet counseling • Preparation and selection of special diets
Health care administrator	• Baccalaureate degree • Master's degree in hospital administration preferred	• Management of health care agency
Occupational therapist	• Baccalaureate degree • Internship for certification	• Promotion and maintenance of activities of daily living • Skill development • Task selection aimed at identified health needs
Pastoral care worker	• Varied • Preparation in pastoral ministry recommended	• Attending to spiritual needs of patient and family
Pharmacist	• Baccalaureate degree • Licensure required	• Preparing and dispensing prescribed medications
Physical therapist	• Baccalaureate degree • Registration	• Promotion of increased muscle strength and mobility
Physician	• Baccalaureate degree • 3–4 yr medical school • Internship and residency required by some states • Licensure required	• Diagnosis and treatment of illness
Registered nurse	• Diploma • Associate degree • Master's or doctor's degree for some positions • Licensure required	• Care at the primary, secondary, and tertiary health levels
Respiratory therapist	• Associate degree • Baccalaureate degree • Optional internship	• Management of pulmonary dysfunction
Social worker	• Baccalaureate degree • Master's degree preferred	• Meeting social needs of individuals, families, and groups

of preparation, with additional study in the philosophy of osteopathy and its application in practice through manipulative therapy. All physicians are required to take a state board licensing examination prior to practice as an MD or DO.

Respiratory Therapist

The **respiratory therapist** evaluates, treats, and cares for clients with respiratory alterations. These therapists assist the client in meeting the oxygen requirements of the body and assist in diagnostic testing of pulmonary dysfunctions. Educational preparation varies, but associate and baccalaureate programs are becoming more popular. A master's degree is required in many positions.

Social Worker

The **social worker** assists clients and families with financial and social problems through utilization of community and government resources. Such activities may include providing emotional support, assisting with living arrangements, and making referrals to community agencies and nursing homes. Education is at the baccalaureate and master's degree level. A master's degree is required for membership in the National Association of Social Workers. A medical social work specialty is available at the master's level.

Table 5–1 summarizes the types of health care providers discussed, the focus of their involvement in health care, and recommended educational preparation.

CULTURAL FOLK PRACTICES AND ALTERNATIVE HEALTH CARE

The previous sections of this chapter deal with the health care delivery system as the formal means of obtaining health care. This section addresses some of the informal means of obtaining health care. **Informal health care** means include "individual cultural beliefs and practices that often occur outside of the formal, established health care delivery system of the majority culture." Within cultures, there may be subcultures with diverse cultural perceptions and expectations of health, health care, and health behavior. The study of culture and health as it relates to nursing care is very complex and diverse. For the nurse to help clients adequately progress toward their own culturally defined health state, it is essential to view clients from the point of view of their own individual cultural beliefs and practices.

Leininger (1967) provides an example of the use of informal means for achieving health and the cultural differences that can occur in relation to reception of health care.

This example occurs in an outpatient clinic where a nursing student, a Mexican-American mother, and her 3-year-old daughter were interacting. The nursing student repeatedly expressed how pretty the young daughter was but never touched the daughter. The student noted that the mother became restless and withdrew from the conversation and interpreted the mother's behavior as a result of a language barrier. The student continued to stress the daughter's beauty to the mother. As soon as the student was called away, the mother left the clinic. Upon arriving home, the mother called her native midwife friends (*parteras*) and related the incident. She explained that she thought the student had cast an evil eye (*mal ojo*) on the daughter. Later the mother talked with a native health practitioner (*curandero*) for additional advice. All believed the child was under malevolent magical forces due to the nursing student's behavior. To confirm the belief, the child's skin was rubbed with the substance from a broken egg, and a red spot appeared. This confirmed that, by complimenting the child without rubbing her head, the student had cast an evil eye on the child. The culturally preferred way to cure the child was to have the responsible person rub the child's head. In this case, the mother was afraid to return to the clinic, so the mother and the native curers treated the child with several methods to counteract the negative forces of the evil eye. Upon hearing of this incident, the student stated that it was not customary in the Anglo-American culture to hold or touch a child without first establishing a relationship with the mother, while in some other cultures it is considered to be an insult to hold or touch a child.

While this is an example of diverse cultural beliefs, there are also examples related specifically to diverse health practices or health beliefs. Powers (1982) offers an example of health practices of some black Americans.

A middle-aged black woman was seen in a health care center for possible heart failure, obesity, and elevated blood pressure. A health care practitioner was to provide instruction on weight reduction and blood pressure management. After instruction and upon subsequent clinic visits, it was determined that no change occurred. When the woman visited the clinic, she always expressed gratitude for the instruction and indicated that the practitioner's instruction was beneficial. The practitioner began including more informal conversation in the visits. It was found that the woman had also been visiting a root doctor who had prescribed a powerful cure. The root doctor was thought to be born with the gift of healing and to be very powerful. The woman felt that someone had put a "root" on her that required someone of equal power (root doctor) to remove. "Treatment tended to involve a religious aspect such as prayer and the burning of candles; a medicinal aspect, such as tea or potion to be prepared following strict specifications; and a magical ritual aspect such as washing a man's shirt in boiling water, carrying it to the river, turning around three times while reciting a given chant and throwing the shirt into the river" (p. 39). More than one root doctor may be necessary for ailments. In hearing of this experience, the practitioner learned that it is important to recollect and examine daily life events in monitoring health and explaining illness. The practitioner then focused on personal interaction, which had more congruence with the woman's folk practices than did the mere giving of instruction.

Hautman & Harrison (1982) describe health beliefs and practices of middle-income Anglo-Americans. Some beliefs held by this group include that viruses and bacteria cause diseases such as measles; "nerves" cause shingles; stress and obesity result in hypertension (high blood pressure); and drafts, cold air, and environmental fluctuations cause colds. Home remedies reported by this group were honey, tea, and lemon for colds; buttermilk for gastric problems; cold tea bags over burned areas followed by vitamin E ointment; mustard plaster for colds; catnip tea for nerves; horehound drops for lung problems; and copper bracelets for arthritis. Some "alternatives to orthodox practices" included chiropractors for bone and back disorders; nutritionists for obesity; and herbalists for various health ailments.

Some of these cultural practices have been incorporated into the formal methods of health care delivery in the United States. Other practices that are gaining more popularity include biofeedback, hypnosis, relaxation, music therapy, imagery, faith healing, acupuncture, touch, and massage. Both formal and informal means of obtaining health care services have been described. Health care professionals must be aware of their own health beliefs as well as the cultural health beliefs of others and provide care that is congruent with these beliefs. Nurses can become involved in the informal health care system by incorporating cultural beliefs of the clients in planned nursing action as well as in community educational programs and private practice.

SUMMARY

The HCDS is an open, interacting system. It has been described in terms of formal and informal means of obtaining health care. The system is undergoing many changes in response to social and financial pressures. The formal means of health care delivery include methods of classifying the system (official or public, voluntary or nonprofit, and proprietary or profit making) and levels of prevention. Major health care services are discussed, and health care providers are described within the context of areas of responsibility. Examples of informal means of obtaining health care are given.

▶ Questions for Discussion

1. How would you explain the health care delivery system to a consumer?
2. A neighbor of yours has recently been a client in various parts of the health delivery system. He expresses concern about the numbers of "different faces" (various health personnel) in the health care system. How would you explain the various health care providers?
3. Describe some informal health care practices followed by you and your family.
4. What are the levels of prevention used in classifying health care delivery? Give some examples.

REFERENCES

Aiken L. Transformation of the nursing workforce. *Nurs Outlook.* 1995; 43:201–209.

Aroskar M. Access to hospice, ethical dimensions. *Nurs Clin North Am.* 1985; 20:299–310.

Center for Disease Control. *Ten leading causes of death in the United States.* Atlanta: CDC; 1994.

Cornett B. Alternative delivery systems: Update for the occupational health nurse. *Occup Health Nurs.* 1984; 32:581–583.

Deeds S. Health-promotion activities in selected HMO settings. *Fam Community Health.* 1985; 8(1):1–17.

Erwin W. AHA survey; nurse shortage eases dramatically. *Hospitals.* 1993; 7(3):52.

Hautman M, Harrison JK. Health: beliefs and practices in a middle income Anglo-American neighborhood. *Adv Nurs Sci.* 1982; 4:281–300.

Holthaus R. Nurse-managed health care: An ongoing tradition. *Nurse Pract Forum.* 1993; 4(3):128–132.

Iglehart J. The American health care system: managed care. In: Philip Lee and Carroll Estes, eds. *The Nation's Health.* 4th ed. Boston: Jones and Bartlett Publishers; 1994.

Knickman J, Thorpe K. Financing health care. In: Kovner A, ed. *Jonas's*

Health Care Delivery in the United States. 5th ed. New York: Springer; 1995:267–293.

Lancaster J, Lancaster W. Current status of the health care system. In: Stanhope M, Lancaster J, eds. *Community Health Nursing Process and Practice for Promoting Health.* St. Louis: Mosby; 1984:32–53.

Leavell HR, Clark EG. *Preventive Medicine for the Doctor in His Community.* New York: McGraw-Hill; 1965.

Leininger M. The culture concept and its relevance to nursing. *J Nurs Educ.* 1967; 6(2):27–37.

Levey S, Loomba NP. *Health Care Administration: A Managerial Perspective.* Philadelphia: Lippincott; 1973.

Levit K, Sensenig A, Cowan C, Lazenby H, McDonnell P, Won D, Sivarajan L, Stiller J, Donham, C, & Stewart M. National health expenditures, 1993. *Health Care Financing Review/*Fall. 1994; 16(1):247–268. USDHHS, HCFA Pub # 03361.

McMahon B, Berlin J. Health of the United States population. In: Lee P, Brown N, Red I, eds. *The Nation's Health.* San Francisco: Boyd and Fraser; 1981.

National HMO Census. *Annual Report on the Growth of HMOs in the United States.* Excelsior, MN: Interstudy; 1983.

National League for Nursing. *Nursing's Agenda for Health Care Reform.* New York: NLN; 1991.

Pender N. *Health Promotion in Nursing Practice.* 3rd ed. Norwalk, CT: Appleton & Lange; 1996.

PEW Health Professions Commission. *Health America. Practitioners for 2005.* PEW Health Commission; 1991.

Powers B. The use of orthodox and black American folk medicine. *Adv Nurs Sci.* 1982; 4(3):35–47.

Relman, A. The health care industry: Where is it taking us? In: Philip Lee and Carroll Estes, eds. *The Nation's Health.* 4th ed. Boston: Jones and Bartlett Publishers; 1994.

Salsberg E, Kovner C. The health care workforce. In: Kovner A, ed. *Jonas's Health Care Delivery in the United States.* 5th ed. New York: Springer; 1995:55–100.

Shamansky S, Clausen C. Levels of prevention: Examination of the concept. *Nurs Outlook.* 1980; 28:104–108.

Stewart J. *Home Health Care.* St. Louis: Mosby; 1979.

Turner JB, ed. *Encyclopedia of Social Work.* Washington, D.C.: National Association of Social Workers; 1977.

U.S. Department of Health and Human Services. *Agency for Health Care Policy and Research.* (AHCPR Pub. # 94–0592). Washington, D.C.: Government Printing Office; 1994.

U.S. Department of Labor. *Labstat Series Reports.* Bureau of Labor Statistics; June 12, 1993.

U.S. Public Health Service. *Healthy People 2000, National Health Promotion and Disease Prevention Objectives.* Washington, D.C.: U.S. Government Printing Office; 1990.

Walker PH. Comprehensive community nursing center. Maximizing practice income: A challenge to education. *J Prof Nurs* 1994; 10:131–139.

Wilson L. The American revolution in health care. *AAOHN J.* 1988; 36:402–407.

Yeaworth RC. Changing perspectives on health care. In: Chaska NL, ed. *The Nursing Profession: A Time to Speak.* New York: McGraw-Hill; 1983: 858–868.

BIBLIOGRAPHY

DeLew N, Greenberg G, Kinchen K. A layman's guide to the U.S. health care system. *Health Care Financ Rev*/Fall. 1992; 14(1):151–169.

Dunham-Taylor J, Marquette P, Pinczuk J. Surviving capitation. *Am J Nurs.* 1996; 96:26–30.

Ellis JR, Hartlay C. *Nursing in Today's World: Challenges, Issues and Trends.* 5th ed. Philadelphia: Lipincott; 1995.

Glittenberg J. Adapting health care to a cultural setting. *Am J Nurs.* 1974; 74:1118.

Hamilton JM. Nursing and DRGs: Proactive responses to prospective reimbursement. *Nurs Health Care.* 1984; 5:155–160.

Joel LA. DRGs: The state of the art of reimbursement of nursing services. *Nurs Health Care.* 1983; 4:560–564.

Kosko D, Flaskerud J. Mexican-American, nurse practitioner, and lay control group beliefs about cause and treatment of chest pain. *Nurs Res.* 1987; 36:226–231.

Lattanzi ME. Hospice bereavement services: Creating networks of support. *Fam Community Health.* 1982; 5(3):54–63.

Moore P, Williamson C. Health promotion evolution of concept. *Nurs Clin North Am.* 1984; 19:195–205.

Richard E. A rationale for incorporating wellness programs into existing occupational health programs. *Occup Health Nurs.* 1984; 32:412–415.

Riley D. International health care systems: Emerging models. *Nurs Econ.* 1994; 12(4):201.

Schroeder L. Nursing's response to the crisis of access, costs, and quality in health care. *Adv Nurs Sci.* 1993; 16(1):1–20.

Shaffer F. A nursing perspective of the DRG world: Part I. *Nurs Health Care.* 1984; 5(1):48–51.

Shaffer F. DRGs: History and overview. *Nurs Health Care.* 1983; 4:388–396.

Sovie M. Tailoring hospitals for managed care and integrated health systems. *Nurs Econ.* 1995; 13(2):72–88.

Stahl D. Integrated delivery system: An opportunity or a dilemma. *Nurs Man.* 1995; 26(7):20–23.

6
CHAPTER

Nursing Practice in Various Settings

▶ **Objectives**

After studying the chapter the student will be able to:

1. Define the components of the nursing process.
2. Discuss the elements of the role of the professional nurse.
3. Identify factors influencing the role of the nurse.
4. Describe the various nursing positions in community and hospital settings.
5. Describe the role of the nurse as it is implemented within various health care settings.
6. Discuss various areas of nursing specialization.
7. Describe several elements of the role used within each practice setting.

▶ **Questions to think about before reading the chapter**

- What is the nursing process?
- How would you describe the role of the nurse?
- In what areas have you seen nurses practice?
- Are you aware of any areas of specialization for nurses? If so, what are they?
- How would the implementation of the role of the nurse in a community setting be the same and how would it differ from a hospital setting?

▶ **Terms to know:**

Advanced practice	Change agent
American Nurses Association (ANA)	Client advocate
Assessment	Collaborator
Caregiver	Consultant

Coordinator

Counselor

Critical thinking

Data

Decision-making

Educator

Evaluation

Goal setting

Hall, Lydia

Implementation

Interpersonal process

North American Nursing Diagnosis
   Association (NANDA)

Nursing care plan

Nursing diagnosis

Nursing Interventions Classification (NIC)

Nurse practitioner

Nursing process

Nursing skills

Objective data

Planning

Practice

Role

Standards of Clinical Nursing Practice

Subjective data

Unlicensed assistive personnel (UAP)

Visiting nurse association

▶ *Introduction*

Opportunities for nursing practice are continually developing. In this chapter, the focus is on critical thinking and the nursing process, the nursing role with its many elements, and the implementation of the elements of the nurse's role as health care provider within the health care delivery system. The practice component of nursing, nursing process, is described as a vehicle for implementation of theory as well as validation and impetus for research. Nursing process is introduced as a framework for decision making, allowing for critical thinking and problem solving when approaching client care. Nursing, like many other practice professions, is not limited to one area of practice. The identification of a client's health care needs provides a variety of opportunities for nurses to implement their role. The role of nursing, however, remains constant in the various practice areas, although the implementation is dynamic, continually changing, and expanding. This chapter discusses various opportunities for nursing practice in the community, hospital, and long-term settings.

Some of these opportunities include nursing in community health settings, occupational health settings, rural settings, clinics, prenatal and well-child centers, schools, offices, private practice, private duty, camps, community mental health agencies, hospices, skilled care facilities, and rehabilitation centers. Included with the discussions are descriptions of these settings, educational requirements, and the functions of nurses within the nursing and health care teams. The final section of the chapter discusses the nurse's role as a health care provider in selected advanced practice arenas including those of the clinical specialist, nurse practitioner, nurse midwife, and nurse anesthetist. In addition, the roles of the nurse in nursing education, nursing administration, and nursing research are discussed.

PRACTICE

Practice is an aspect of nursing that incorporates both science (e.g., biology, chemistry, anatomy) and the arts and humanities (e.g., sociology, language, psychology) into its practice. The practice aspect of nursing has been defined by many sources within the profession itself and also by societal sources.

Within the profession, nurses as individuals or as groups have defined practice. For example, individual nurses have described nursing as enhancing the strengths of the individual by viewing the total person. The physical, psychological, cultural, spiritual, and social aspects are considered in helping the person respond as normally as possible to life situations. The **American Nurses Association (ANA)** is the professional nursing organization contributing to the definition of nursing practice.

In 1991 the ANA published *Standards of Clinical Nursing Practice,* which focuses on care provided to all clients including individuals, families, groups, or communities. It addresses care that "may be provided in the context of disease or injury prevention, health promotion, health restoration, or health maintenance." The Standards take into account culture, race, and ethnic diversity. The Standards consist of "Standards of Care" and "Standards of Professional Performance." With increased personal and professional growth in nursing, nurses have developed an increased awareness of the need to assume responsibility for actions by the profession. Therefore, the standards of practice that have been developed by the ANA enhance nursing autonomy and accountability. The general standards of clinical practice follow:

Standards of Care

- Standard I. Assessment
  The nurse collects client health data.
- Standard II. Diagnosis
  The nurse analyzes the assessment data in determining diagnoses.

- Standard III. Outcome Identification
  The nurse identifies expected outcomes individualized to the client.
- Standard IV. Planning
  The nurse develops a plan of care that prescribes interventions to attain expected outcomes.
- Standard V. Implementation
  The nurse implements the interventions identified in the plan of care.
- Standard VI. Evaluation
  The nurse evaluates the client's progress toward attainment of outcomes.

Standards of Professional Performance

- Standard I. Quality of Care
  The nurse systematically evaluates the quality and effectiveness of nursing practice.
- Standard II. Performance Appraisal
  The nurse evaluates his or her own nursing practice in relation to professional practice standards and relevant statutes and regulations.
- Standard III. Education
  The nurse acquires and maintains current knowledge in nursing practice.
- Standard IV. Collegiality
  The nurse contributes to the professional development of peers, colleagues, and others.
- Standard V. Ethics
  The nurse's decisions and actions on behalf of clients are determined in an ethical manner.
- Standard VI. Collaboration
  The nurse collaborates with the client, significant others, and health care providers in providing client care.
- Standard VII. Research
  The nurse uses research findings in practice.
- Standard VIII. Resource Utilization
  The nurse considers factors related to safety, effectiveness, and cost in planning and delivering client care.

Through the interaction of nursing with society, nursing practice changes and nursing is challenged to address societal health needs. While the implementation of the role of the nurse changes under the influence of such factors as scientific developments, legislation, legal issues, and technology, practice is based on nursing's theoretical concepts. In return, practice generates further research for nursing. An example of the interactive process of nursing and society is that of the legislative and legal system and the formation of individual state nurse practice acts. Nurse practice acts govern the scope of nursing and exist primarily to assure minimally safe nursing care to members of society. Nurses serve as lobbyists to ensure that nursing is represented throughout the legal process. Each state has a board of nursing appointed by the governor of that state. These nursing boards are responsible for the implementation and regulation of the practice acts. Other changes in health care and nursing practice that have been influenced by society are informed consent, advocacy, accountability, men in the profession, and women's rights.

Along with these changes, nursing skills have expanded to include health assessment, interpersonal relations, technical and cognitive skills, use of teaching-learning principles, and research methodology. These skills are practiced with individual clients, groups, families, and communities. Nursing is a dynamic profession as practice, theory, and research continue to evolve. Contemporary roles of the professional nurse have continued to develop and are discussed later in this chapter. One of the changes occurring in nursing practice has been the evolution of a systematic process for nursing care. This process has been labeled *the nursing process.*

NURSING PROCESS

In the literature, processes, or ways in which something is done, are frequently discussed. The use of a process in decision-making situations contributes to efficiency and accuracy. The following situation depicts the benefits of using a process in **decision-making.** A high school senior is planning for the future and considering options. He begins by collecting information. Subjectively (from his own perspective) he may identify some of the following:

- "I am interested in college."
- "I like to study."
- "People really interest me, and I would like to help them."
- "I feel able to meet the requirements."
- "I might be homesick, but I think I can adjust."

Objectively (from the perspective of others) the student may identify:

- Other people have told him that he has the potential for college work and that he would be empathetic in patient situations.

- His high school grade point average is 3.0. College test scores place him in the 90th percentile.
- He has $5000.00 in savings and has a job for the summer.

After the information or **data** are reflected on together, they are given meaning, or interpreted, by searching out available information on college. For instance, the student may gather information on a particular field or discipline such as nursing. The data are then interpreted by the student, comparing the requirements for entrance into a college nursing program with his own qualifications. From interpretation of the data, the student can make a decision, or judgment, to go to college. For example: The student has shown evidence of his potential for college nursing education. If a decision were made without such a process, that is, if it were based on intuition, it would likely be far less accurate.

Once a decision is made, there is a basis for **goal setting,** an action that also involves process. The student has identified a personal potential for college nursing education and now needs to identify what existing programs are suited to his particular circumstances. One of the many goals in meeting this need might be to obtain information on collegiate schools of nursing by January. Information would be obtained by following a plan, such as looking up collegiate schools of nursing in the library, writing to each of the schools for information, and visiting those identified as most suited to his needs. Finally, achievement of goals would need to be evaluated. For instance, in January he would evaluate the extent to which useful information has been gathered. Thus, process is essential to accurate decision making and goal-directed activities.

Nursing also uses a process that forms the framework and integrating component for carrying on its activities (practice). The nursing process is a deliberative, systematic approach to nursing care based on scientific inquiry and problem-solving methods. Through the use of the process, the nurse generates information concerning patient care situations and contributes to the body of knowledge of nursing (theory). The nurse draws from a body of knowledge to validate the findings in client care situations. Through the use of the process, questions are posed and ideas are generated regarding clients, their health, the effects of the environment on health, and the effects of nursing care in contributing to health. These questions and ideas form the basis of clinical nursing inquiry (research).

Nursing process as it is known today evolved as nursing itself evolved. As early as 1955, **Lydia Hall** spoke of the need for a formalized process. In 1967, a committee of the western states defined nursing process within the framework of interpersonal process. In the same year, at Catholic University, nursing process was defined as assessment, planning, implementation, and evaluation. These later became the steps of nursing process, and each step became more clearly defined (Yura & Walsh, 1988). Many nursing theorists have defined nursing process within their conceptual models. Table 6–1 summarizes these definitions.

Nursing process is an integrating component for the provision of nursing care and describes the clinical decision-making process used in the identification, planning, implementation, and evaluation of nursing care. Nursing, as a learned profession, bases its practice on systematically gathered information and a complete data base. The nursing process gives direction, order, accountability, and responsibility to nursing practice. Theories and concepts from science and the humanities and arts are applied in practice through the use of nursing process. It is a systematic and dynamic process, designed to help nurses facilitate client achievement and maintenance of health, as well as to improve the quality of care. Through the use of process, the nurse's care is based on the individual needs of the client, family, or group rather than on routine tasks. Like the student who followed a process in decision making for college entrance, the nurse using a process increases the probability of accurate decision making for client care.

Many skills are needed when using the nursing process including: **critical thinking,** problem solving, decision-making, interper-

TABLE 6–1. SUMMARY OF DEFINITIONS OF NURSING PROCESS BY NURSING AUTHORS

Name	Nursing Process
Hildegard Peplau	Phases of nurse–patient relationship; four interlocking phases: orientation, exploration, identification, and resolution
Ernestine Wiedenbach	Delineates interrelation and interdependence of knowledge, judgment, and skills to meet patient needs for help; identification, administration, validation of help needed, and coordination of resources
Virginia Henderson	Deliberative, individual care involving assessing, planning, and evaluating the individual using the 14 components
Dorothy Johnson	Four models of intervention involving drive, set, choice, and action; goals
Dorothea Orem	Involves diagnosis, prescription, treatment, and management of care
Imogene King	Goal attainment is the basis for the nursing process. Process is the interaction between client and nurse to set goals and agree upon means to achieve them
Sr. Callista Roy	Assessment, diagnosis, goal setting, and intervention are the components of the process. Intervention involves manipulating the focal, contextual, and residual stimuli
Martha Rogers	Not explicated in this model

sonal skills, and technical skills. The process can be applied to individuals, families, groups, and communities and is the basis for contemporary nursing.

Yura and Walsh (1988) describe the nursing process as central to all nursing actions, applicable in any setting, within any theoretical conceptual reference. It is described as flexible, adaptable, and adjustable to a number of variables. Bandman and Bandman (1995) describe the process as a means to demonstrate accountability for nursing care. The process can provide a framework for the implementation of the various roles of the nurse.

Nursing education emphasizes the nursing process as a method of approaching client care, since the process encompasses theory, practice, and research. The nursing process is used extensively as one of the core concepts in nursing education.

Nursing process may be described as having eight characteristics:

1. It is a cognitive process.
2. It is client-centered.
3. It is goal-directed.
4. It is planned.
5. It involves a series of steps.
6. It is a circular and cyclical process.
7. Its phases are sequential.
8. All phases must be included and are often overlapping.

The phases in nursing process illustrated in Figure 6–1 are very similar to the phases identified in the process example previously cited. The actual steps of the nursing process are:

1. Assessment.
2. Analysis and nursing diagnosis.
3. Planning.
4. Implementation.
5. Evaluation.

Assessment, the first phase of the nursing process, consists of the collection of subjective and objective data about the health care status of a client. **Subjective data** is information obtained directly from the client through interviews. It is what the client thinks or experiences that cannot be seen by others. **Objective data** is factual information obtained through the use of the assessor's senses. The data are collected by means of an organized data-gathering tool adapted to the situation. An initial assessment is completed on first contact with the client. Ongoing assessments are made on a regular basis while the client is receiving nursing care. Some information categories that may be used in an initial data assessment include:

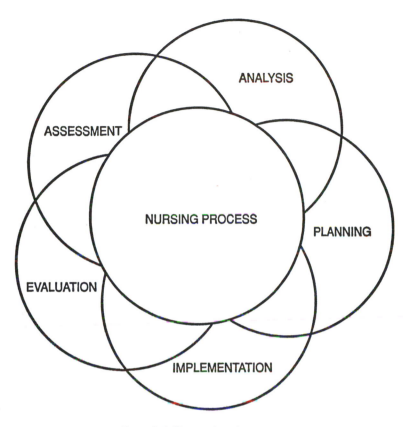

Figure 6–1. Phases of nursing process.

I. Nursing history
   A. General information (age, sex, height, weight)
   B. Past and present health history (self and family)
   C. Perceptions of health and illness
   D. Perceived current and long-term effects of illness and treatment
   E. Activities of daily living (mobility, nutrition, sleep, elimination, and self-care)
   F. Socioeconomic status
   G. Education
   H. Religion and spirituality
   I. Family interactional patterns
   J. Review of health status of body systems
II. Physical Examination
   A. Head and neck
   B. Thorax
   C. Abdomen

    D. Skin and extremities
    E. Genitalia
    F. Neurological

From the data collected, significant data are grouped together and interpreted in terms of principles, concepts, theories, and research. A variety of methods are used to organize nursing data including human needs, human response patterns, body systems, and functional patterns. A method in common use, which employs a topology of human functional patterns, is described by Gordon (1987). These patterns enable the nurse to organize data about the client in order to make a clinical judgment. No matter what method is used, once a comprehensive data base is obtained and interpreted, the nurse analyzes the information and makes a decision as to the health status or actual or potential needs or problems, "which nurses by virtue of their education and experience are capable and licensed to treat." This clinical judgment is currently being labeled a **nursing diagnosis** (Gordon, 1976, p. 1299).

"Nursing diagnoses provide the basis for selection of nursing interventions to achieve outcomes for which the nurse is accountable" (9th conference of NANDA). Carpenito (1995) describes four types of nursing diagnoses. Actual diagnosis describes a validated clinical judgment because of the presence of major defining characteristics, risk diagnosis describes a clinical judgment based on an individual's vulnerability to develop a particular problem, wellness diagnosis is a clinical judgment about the level of wellness of an individual or group, syndrome diagnosis is a cluster of actual or risk "nursing diagnoses that are predicted to present because of a certain situation or event" (p. xxvi). The diagnostic statement usually consists of the statement of health status and the contributing factors. The nursing diagnosis should be validated through client feedback whenever possible.

Nursing diagnoses are not new. In 1973, efforts began to identify, standardize, and classify health problems treated by nurses at the First National Conference on Classification of Nursing Diagnoses. Since that conference in 1973, conferences have been held on a biennial basis. In 1982, the conference renamed the association the **North American Nursing Diagnosis Association (NANDA)**. From the work of the association, a taxonomy of nine patterns of human responses was developed. This taxonomy is used as a classification system that is followed by two or more levels that are more concrete and applicable to the practitioner. These levels include diagnostic labels or statements. Table 6–2 lists the nursing diagnoses currently accepted by NANDA by their classification number. The list of nursing diagnoses developed for testing is under continual revision and

TABLE 6–2. NANDA NURSING DIAGNOSES CLASSIFICATION

Pattern 1: Exchanging

1.1.2.1	Altered Nutrition: More than Body Requirements
1.1.2.2	Altered Nutrition: Less than Body Requirements
1.1.2.3	Altered Nutrition: Potential for More than Body Requirements
1.2.1.1	Risk for Infection
1.2.2.1	Risk for Altered Body Temperature
1.2.2.2	Hypothermia
1.2.2.3	Hyperthermia
1.2.2.4	Ineffective Thermoregulation
1.2.3.1	Dysreflexia
1.3.1.1	Constipation
1.3.1.1.1	Perceived Constipation
1.3.1.1.2	Colonic Constipation
1.3.1.2	Diarrhea
1.3.1.3	Bowel Incontinence
1.3.2	Altered Urinary Elimination
1.3.2.1.1	Stress Incontinence
1.3.2.1.2	Reflex Incontinence
1.3.2.1.3	Urge Incontinence
1.3.2.1.4	Functional Incontinence
1.3.2.1.5	Total Incontience
1.3.2.2	Urinary Retention
1.4.1.1	Altered (specify type) Tissue Perfusion (renal, cerebral, cardiopulmonary, gastrointestinal, peripheral)
1.4.1.2.1	Fluid Volume Excess
1.4.1.2.2.1	Fluid Volume Deficit
1.4.1.2.2.2	Risk for Fluid Volume Deficit
1.4.2.1	Decreased Cardiac Output
1.5.1.1	Impaired Gas Exchange
1.5.1.2	Ineffective Airway Clearance
1.5.1.3	Ineffective Breathing Pattern
1.5.1.3.1	Inability to Sustain Spontaneous Ventilation
1.5.1.3.2	Dysfunctional Ventilatory Weaning Response (DVWR)
1.6.1	Risk for Injury
1.6.1.1	Risk for Suffocation
1.6.1.2	Risk for Poisoning
1.6.1.3	Risk for Trauma
1.6.1.4	Risk for Aspiration
1.6.1.5	Risk for Disuse Syndrome
1.6.2	Altered Protection
1.6.2.1	Impaired Tissue Integrity
1.6.2.1.1	Altered Oral Mucous Membrane
1.6.2.1.2.1	Impaired Skin Integrity
1.6.2.1.2.2	Risk for Impaired Skin Integrity
1.7.1	Decreased Adaptive Capacity: Intracranial
1.8	Energy Field Disturbance

Pattern 2: Communicating

2.1.1.1	Impaired Verbal Communication

(*continued*)

TABLE 6–2. NANDA NURSING DIAGNOSES CLASSIFICATION (*CONTINUED*)

Pattern 3: Relating

3.1.1	Impaired Social Interaction
3.1.2	Social Isolation
3.1.3	Risk for Loneliness
3.2.1	Altered Role Performance
3.2.1.1.1	Altered Parenting
3.2.1.1.2	Risk for Altered Parenting
3.2.1.1.2.1	Risk for Altered Parent/Infant/Child Attachment
3.2.1.2.1	Sexual Dysfunction
3.2.2	Altered Family Processes
3.2.2.1	Caregiver Role Strain
3.2.2.2	Risk for Caregiver Role Strain
3.2.2.3.1	Altered Family Process: Alcoholism
3.2.3.1	Parental Role Conflict
3.3	Altered Sexuality Patterns

Pattern 4: Valuing

4.1.1	Spiritual Distress (Distress of the Human Spirit)
4.2	Potential for Enhanced Spiritual Well-Being

Pattern 5: Choosing

5.1.1.1	Ineffective Individual Coping
5.1.1.1.1	Impaired Adjustment
5.1.1.1.2	Defensive Coping
5.1.1.1.3	Ineffective Denial
5.1.2.1.1	Ineffective Family Coping: Disabling
5.1.2.1.2	Ineffective Family Coping: Compromised
5.1.2.2	Family Coping: Potential for Growth
5.1.3.1	Potential for Enhanced Community Coping
5.1.3.2	Ineffective Community Coping
5.2.1	Ineffective Management of Therapeutic Regimen (individuals)
5.2.1.1	Noncompliance (specify)
5.2.2	Ineffective Management of Therapeutic Regimen: Families
5.2.3	Ineffective Management of Therapeutic Regimen: Community
5.2.4	Effective Management of Therapeutic Regimen: Individual
5.3.1.1	Decisional Conflict (specify)
5.4	Health-Seeking Behaviors (specify)

Pattern 6: Moving

6.1.1.1	Impaired Physical Mobility
6.1.1.1.1	Risk for Peripheral Neurovascular Dysfunction
6.1.1.1.2	Risk for Perioperative Positioning Injury
6.1.1.2	Activity Intolerance
6.1.1.2.1	Fatigue
6.1.1.3	Risk for Activity Intolerance
6.2.1	Sleep Pattern Disturbance
6.3.1.1	Diversional Activity Deficit
6.4.1.1	Impaired Home Maintenance Management
6.4.2	Altered Health Maintenance

TABLE 6–2. NANDA NURSING DIAGNOSES CLASSIFICATION (*CONTINUED*)

6.5.1	Feeding Self-Care Deficit
6.5.1.1	Impaired Swallowing
6.5.1.2	Ineffective Breast Feeding
6.5.1.2.1	Interrupted Breast Feeding
6.5.1.3	Effective Breast Feeding
6.5.1.4	Ineffective Infant Feeding Pattern
6.5.2	Bathing/Hygiene Self-Care Deficit
6.5.3	Dressing/Grooming Self-Care Deficit
6.5.4	Toileting Self-Care Deficit
6.6	Altered Growth and Development
6.7	Relocation Stress Syndrome
6.8.1	Risk for Disorganized Infant Behavior
6.8.2	Disorganized Infant Behavior
6.8.3	Potential for Enhanced Organized Infant Behavior

Pattern 7: Perceiving

7.1.1	Body Image Disturbance
7.1.2	Self-Esteem Disturbance
7.1.2.1	Chronic Low Self-Esteem
7.1.2.2	Situational Low Self-Esteem
7.1.3	Personal Identity Disturbance
7.2	Sensory/Perceptual Alterations (specify) (visual, auditory, kinesthetic, gustatory, tactile, olfactory)
7.2.1.1	Unilateral Neglect
7.3.1	Hopelessness
7.3.2	Powerlessness

Pattern 8: Knowing

8.1.1	Knowledge Deficit (specify)
8.2.1	Impaired Environmental Interpretation Syndrome
8.2.2	Acute Confusion
8.2.3	Chronic Confusion
8.3	Altered Throught Processes
8.3.1	Impaired Memory

Pattern 9: Feeling

9.1.1	Pain
9.1.1.1	Chronic Pain
9.2.1.1	Dysfunctional Grieving
9.2.1.2	Anticipatory Grieving
9.2.2	Risk for Violence: Self-Directed or Directed at Others
9.2.2.1	Risk for Self-Mutilation
9.2.3	Post-Trauma Response
9.2.3.1	Rape-Trauma Syndrome
9.2.3.1.1	Rape-Trauma Syndrome: Compound Reaction
9.2.3.1.2	Rape-Trauma Syndrome: Silent Reaction
9.3.1	Anxiety
9.3.2	Fear

subject to validation through research. Nurses in psychiatric and mental health care are developing nursing diagnoses to specifically address patterns of psychosocial behavior. Nursing diagnoses other than those formally established are also being used by nurses and are requested by NANDA for review and possible adoption. In addition to the review of new diagnoses, currently accepted diagnoses are also reviewed for applicability to current practice. Some may be too broad, others too specific to address the current health needs of the client (Carpenito, 1995).

Some nursing writers disagree with the diagnostic categories, since these categories focus more on client actual or potential health problems and do not adequately address the client holistically, emphasizing client health assets and strengths (Adam, 1991).

Once a nursing diagnosis has been identified, a nursing care plan with specific client-centered objectives or goals and accompanying actions is established. Client goals and criteria are established to direct nursing care. The client-centered goals established for meeting client needs determine the outcome criteria. For example, it may be determined by the nurse and a new father and mother that the parents have a potential for altered parenting related to knowledge deficit secondary to infant care.

The nurse collaborates with the client to establish goals that address the health state or meet the need or problem. It is the responsibility of the nurse to implement the plan of care or direct the implementation.

Nursing skills interventions are used in carrying out specific nursing care activities that may include assisting clients with basic needs; promoting and restoring health; observing and evaluating client response and adaptation to treatment and illness; teaching self-care practices; and counseling and planning goals with clients aimed at self-actualization.

Recent authors have begun to describe and classify independent nursing interventions (Bulechek & McCloskey 1992, and Snyder, 1992). McCloskey and Bulechek (1996) define a nursing intervention as "any treatment, based upon clinical judgment and knowledge, that a nurse performs to enhance patient–client outcomes. Nursing interventions include both direct and indirect care; both nurse-initiated, physician-initiated, and other provider-initiated treatments" (p. xvii).

The **Nursing Interventions Classification (NIC)** was created in the early 1990s to help practitioners document their care, help with standardizing language (nomenclature) of nursing treatments, provide a linkage between nursing diagnoses, treatments, and outcomes, expand nursing knowledge, develop information systems, teach decision making to students, determine cost of services provided by nurses, and to articulate with other health care providers (McCloskey & Bulechek, 1996).

Evaluation is the final phase of the nursing process and is used to determine whether the goals were attained and the plan of care, with accompanying actions, was effective in meeting the client's needs. The nurse, using the nursing process, facilitates the client's decision-making process and assists the client in becoming involved with his or her own care.

Outcome or product evaluation, as it relates to nursing care, reflects on the actual behaviors or responses of the person after a plan of care has been completed. In process evaluation, nursing actions are examined. Examples of the nursing process and its components are shown in the following situation.

Client Situation

A nurse is working at a college student health center and a student enters the center with several complaints of abdominal upset, not feeling well, unable to sleep, and trouble concentrating on course work. The students states "I've never been away from home before, my phone bills are high, and I miss my family. I'm also having trouble with my roommate." The nurse uses the nursing process in the following manner.

Assessment

The nurse uses assessment skills to collect subjective and objective data (information by observation, interview, and interaction).

Data: Student verbal comments (listed above), crying during the interview, eyes tearful with dark circles, hair unkempt.

The data are grouped and interpreted in a meaningful way.

Analysis and Nursing Diagnosis

Through investigation the nurse analyzes the meaning of each piece of data. For example, crying, abdominal upset, inability to sleep may be a physiological response to a situation that is beyond the individual's control.

Analysis leads to one or more nursing diagnoses. One possible nursing diagnosis from the NANDA grouping is "ineffective individual coping related to change in availability of support systems."

Planning

Next, goals that are mutually acceptable to the client when possible are established and a course of action is planned to meet the goals. The goals are always aimed at meeting stated needs and are prioritized. A goal for this client could be "Client will have effective individual coping as evidenced by: a) statement such as 'I am able to focus on my studies more' within 2 weeks; b) during the next interview of the client will not have evidence of crying; c) statement by client 'I was able to sleep all night' or 'my stomach is no longer upset the way it was'."

Actions to attain these goals is directed at using facilitative questions by the nurse to explore strategies with the student to seek out new support systems. Support system enhancement could be selected as an appropriate nursing intervention. Specific activities might include: determining support systems currently being used, determining barriers to using support systems, encouraging relationships with persons who have common interests and goals.

Implementation

The nurse then carries out the actions to achieve the stated goals, thus meeting the client's needs.

Evaluation

The nurse evaluates the goals to see if the desired outcome has been achieved. Behaviors such as no further evidence of crying, statements indicating sleeping throughout the night, or lack of abdominal upset would indicate that goals have been met.

As exemplified in this situation, nursing process is a systematic method of identifying areas for nursing intervention. Nursing process involves the stages of assessment, analysis and nursing diagnosis, **planning, implementation,** and evaluation. Nursing process is based on a scientific foundation and is essential to nursing practice.

ROLE OF THE NURSE

The **practice** of professional nursing is based on theory that is validated and expanded through research and strives to meet the health needs of individuals, families, groups, and society. In their role, professional nurses use theory and research to enhance their practice as they provide comfort, ensure safety, and promote health and wellness.

The composition and definition of the **role** of the nurse are common topics of discussion in nursing. Even though consumers of health care have definite expectations of nurses, they remain unclear as to the role of the nurse. Quite frequently *role* is defined in terms of functions or duties, but this can put limits or constraints on nursing, since it dictates specifics rather than viewing the role of nursing in a broader sense. For instance, some people may consider administering medications as the role of the nurse. This is really a function of a larger component of the role of the nurse, the caregiver.

The nurse is responsible for many aspects of client care and involvement. Each institution and nursing setting may specify certain functions the nurse must carry out. For example, hospitals generally require a registered nurse (RN) to be the leader of the nursing team and coordinate nursing care. However, not all nurses within or outside the hospital setting perform all the same functions. Yet they all have a basic role or framework within which to practice nursing.

Fundamental to the understanding of the role of the nurse is an understanding of the concept of role. Role is a goal-directed activity or behavior that is considered acceptable to the culture or given situation (Brooks, Kleine-Krachl, 1983; Leddy & Pepper 1993). The literature emphasizes that, as familiar as the concept of role seems to be, there is striking diversity in its meaning. There are certain prevalent commonalities of role theory. Roles have behavioral references concerned with standards of expected behavior or judgments about behaviors. They reflect goals, values, and sentiments operating in a given situation (Conley, 1974, p. 25). Roles involve individuals in social locations behaving with reference to these expectations as well as to their own feelings. A role involves an action of an individual in a particular setting with some identified expectations. For example, persons applying for a job will behave in a manner consistent with their own expectations as well as what is believed to be the expectations of the employer. To take another example, personal and employer expectations may be met by the nurse providing client teaching in a variety of settings. Role is independent of the holder.

In a much more complex way, these concepts apply to nursing. Because of the social nature of nursing, people have different concepts and expectations of the role of the nurse. For example, a client may expect one set of behaviors from a nurse, such as those in the area of safety and comfort. Families may expect knowledge and understanding of the situation the family member is experiencing. The physician may expect another set of behaviors, such as carrying out prescribed orders. Other allied health professionals (social worker, physical therapist, health care administrators) expect still another set of behaviors from the nurse, such as the facilitation of referrals for social work or physical therapy or the use of administrative abilities for administration. Finally, nurses themselves have their own individual role expectations related to the ability to implement nursing process in direct nursing care and in identifying individual needs in care given to families and clients. Inherent in nursing as a discipline and profession is the responsibility of nurses to interpret these various societal expectations within the framework of nursing theory and research. From these interpretations, the role of the nurse is defined and implemented for practice.

The unavoidable lack of consensus concerning expectations of a role leads to a type of role conflict. The problems of role conflict in nursing are various. One area is the already discussed conflict that occurs as a result of differing expectations of groups outside nursing to which nurses must respond. There also are conflict factors related to roles within nursing groups. For example, some groups of nurses disagree as to what should constitute the role of the professional nurse, e.g., nurses' involvement in health education. Should this be a part of the role of all nurses or a function of specialized nurses? Conflict may arise not only because of the policies of instituting certain aspects of the role but also from the feelings evoked about dealing with these aspects. In the example involving the nurse as educator, a nurse may agree that education is part of the role; however, the nurse may hesitate to educate because of lack of knowledge, anger and anxiety from a perceived lack of time, or the increased responsibility in carrying out this part of the role. The challenge to the profession with regard to role conflict is to continue to develop and maintain integration of the members of the nursing discipline with one another as well as with the group as a whole.

Position, another term in role theory, refers to a particular location within a system. Examples of position in nursing are a director within a community health agency or staff nurse in a hospital setting. The nurse in various positions is in an integral relationship with all other health professionals, including other nurses, as well as with the family and clients. Closely related to position is status, or power. Power can be acquired through personal influence or by assuming a particular position. Positions have varying degrees of power. For instance, a dean of a school of nursing has more power because of the position than the faculty in many administrative decisions. Faculty may have more power than the dean in curriculum decisions. There is individual power and there is group power. Although nurses are the largest professional group, there have been significant social, political, and economic factors that have prevented nurses from achieving their potential status as a powerful group

Elements of the Role of the Nurse

In spite of the differences in the role of the nurse resulting from social pressures within and outside nursing, some elements or aspects remain constant. These are diagrammed in Figure 6–2. The role elements differ from nursing functions. Functions can change from setting to setting; however, the elements are constant and utilized over and over. The elements of the nurse's role include caregiver, client

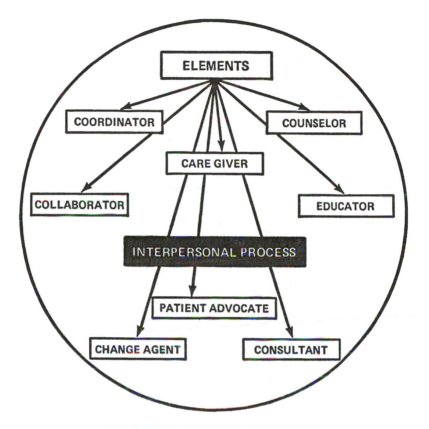

Figure 6–2. Role elements of the professional nurse.

advocate, counselor, educator, coordinator, collaborator, consultant, and change agent. The role elements are implemented within the framework of nursing process.

An interesting method for discussing these elements is through an actual nursing case study, which can be used to describe the elements and their interrelatedness.

A 74-year-old widow, the client, lives alone in a one-bedroom apartment in a federally subsidized housing unit. Her son and daughter live in a nearby community and visit her once every 3 to 4 weeks. The client states that it is difficult to prepare meals and do the grocery shopping. She is on a fixed income and does not have any extra savings. She has been taking a prescribed diuretic to help control blood pressure by increasing systemic fluid excretion (urine output). When transportation is available, the woman has weekly social contacts at her church.

Two day ago, the family physician had to be contacted because of persistent nausea, vomiting, diarrhea, and lack of appetite for several days. The client was admitted to the local community hospital for evaluation. She has been assigned a primary nurse. The responsibility of the nurse is to use nursing process in identifying the health state, or actual or potential problems, of the client. From identified nursing diagnoses, a plan of care is developed.

Caregiver

The first constant element in the perceived role of the nurse, and probably the one most commonly associated with nursing, is that of **caregiver.** As caregiver, the nurse views individuals within the context of their life situations and their significant others. In this element of the role, the nurse uses the nursing process to assess the client's health status and identify nursing diagnoses that may reflect physical, spiritual, cultural, and psychosocial states or needs.

In this case, the client may have a potential alteration in skin integrity related to immobility, and altered nutritional status. The nurse might assess the client for intact skin over bony prominences, food and fluid intake, and ability to move in bed. Measuring a client's temperature, pulse, respiration, and fluid output are other means nurses employ as caregivers to support assessment and evaluation of the client's status. A plan of care for the client may include nursing measures such as removing causative agents and monitoring client status. For instance, the nurse would assist the client to turn every 1 to 2 hours, assess skin integrity, employ devices to reduce skin pressure, massage areas of potential breakdown to stimulate circulation, offer ice chips or small amounts of tolerated fluids. Food likes and dislikes need to be considered. Physical care presumes cognitive and psychomotor skills.

The caregiver element also extends into the psychosocial and spiritual realm. Assisting the client with verbal expression of concerns is an example of a psychosocial measure to alleviate the discomfort of anxiety related to a new environment and her health state. The nurse orients her to the new surroundings to alleviate the anxiety. A physical measure used to alleviate anxiety may be giving a back rub. Spiritual needs may become more evident for persons during illness. As part of the caregiver element, the nurse assesses spiritual needs and includes meeting these needs in planning care. Often the quality of client care is influenced by the caring attitude of the nurse to the client. Nursing care of this client also includes emotional care and support for the client's family.

Client Advocate

Prior to, during, and following hospitalization or an illness episode the client will have contact with many health care providers. As **client advocate,** it is the nurse's responsibility to assist the client and family in interpreting information from other health care providers and in providing additional information needed to make decisions concerning health care. The client advocate element also involves defending and protecting the client's rights.

In the case study, the nurse would support the client during hospitalization for the purpose of receiving increased fluids through intravenous therapy. The client undergoing prolonged hospitalization and intravenous therapy may have a sense of powerlessness. The plan of care for the diagnosis of powerlessness related to perceived loss of control of daily activities may include opportunities for the client to control decisions and manipulate the environment when possible. In addition, the client might determine the schedule for the day's activities.

In a broader context, the nurse may be involved in establishing and implementing institutional policies related to client rights, such as surgical informed consent forms. In our case study, the nurse may have to approach appropriate administrators concerning the client's right to involvement in decision making regarding flexibility of care.

Counselor

Closely related to the patient advocate role element is the element of **counselor**. As a counselor, the nurse first identifies the client's patterns of interaction in dealing with health and illness. Dysfunctional or potentially dysfunctional health patterns are identified, and methods for establishing health-promoting patterns are planned and instituted. The nurse as a counselor may allow the client to express concerns in order to work through feelings and maintain healthy functioning. Counseling serves to aid the person and family in integrating the health experiences with other life experiences.

In the case study presented, the nurse helps the client to identify patterns of social interaction that are not health promoting. For instance, it is noted that the client has diminished social contact with others in her building and at church. The nursing diagnosis may be social isolation related to impaired mobility. A variety of nursing measures may be used by the nurse to help the client solve the problem of reestablishing social contacts. Family members may be consulted concerning the effects of their infrequent visits with the client, always considering their needs and feelings as well as those of the client.

Educator

The **educator** element is employed with client, family, and other health care workers; educating may be incidental (spontaneous at the time of interaction) or formal (preplanned). As an educator, the nurse helps clients promote health through providing knowledge of health-promoting activities, disease-related conditions, and specific treatments. The nursing process is used to determine specific teaching needs of the patient and nursing interventions to meet these needs. Through the educative process clients are helped to become responsible for their own health. Family members and significant others are helped to assume responsibilities for those unable to do so themselves. As the population continues to live longer, education on dealing with chronic health problems has become a priority. The consumer movement and focus on self-care has also increased the demand for health-promoting information.

The client in our case study may have an identified knowledge deficit related to lifestyle following discharge from the hospital. Both incidental and formal discharge teaching may be used to eliminate the knowledge deficit. Incidental teaching might occur after the client is informed that she will be discharged home and followed by a community health nurse. When she asks, "Who will help me with my meals?" the nurse explains what foods are easy to prepare and nutritious, taking into consideration her economic status, living situation, age, and past eating habits. The nurse might also explain the need for replacement of fluids and nutrients. Consideration is also given to the client's anxiety related to meal preparation. If the nurse were to institute a formal teaching plan, optimum time, place, and methods and content of presentation such as educational media would be included. The client could benefit from formal education regarding a balanced diet, environmental influences on food and eating habits, and their relation to health. This formal teaching could be coordinated with advice from the dietitian to provide optimal information and care for the client

Coordinator

Clients receive care from a variety of health care professionals and nonprofessionals. The nurse as a **coordinator** directs, plans, and organizes the care given to the client by the various health team members. Continuing with the client in the case study, the community health nurse would coordinate the efforts of all the health team members in meeting the client's health goals. For example, as a coordinator, the nurse will ensure that the client receives all the necessary professional services to meet her nutritional needs. Two of the professionals working to meet these needs are the dietitian, who assists in meal planning, food preparation, and education regarding food and nutrition; and the social worker, who assists the client with community services such as Meals on Wheels. The nurse participates in health team conferences to facilitate communication among the team, evaluate services given, and plan for continued care.

Collaborator

The **collaborator** element involves the nurse, the client, the family, and other health professionals working together to meet an identified health care need. It involves a sharing of ideas about health care needs, providing support of other professionals, and blending of expertise and skills. Essential to collaboration is the inclusion of family members in the plan of care.

For instance, the community nurse in this case study might collaborate with the physician, the dietitian, and the client in meeting the client's nutritional needs. Together they can develop a plan for diet therapy, including a specialized diet, nutritional supplements, and oral intake. The client may find it difficult to accept a modified diet as part of the plan of care. Helping her accept this involves the supportive relationship of both the physician and the nurse in presenting the plan of care to the client.

Consultant

The **consultant** element implies that individuals involved in client care seek information regarding clarification of patient goals and means of attaining these goals. It also means that the nurse serves as a resource to other health professionals and persons in providing pertinent information about health and nursing care for a specific client situation.

Before discharge, the community health nurse assigned to the client in the case study might consult with the primary nurse in the hospital regarding the client's identified health needs and her limitations and expectations. The client's family might consult with the community nurse regarding their responsibilities in the care. They are included in the assessment of the client and the client situation by the community nurse and may ask the community nurse for this assessment of the client's abilities on discharge and about any special care that may be needed.

Change Agent

The **change agent** element involves planned, collaborative, systematic change in relation to the client, family, populations of clients, and health care delivery services. These health care delivery services may include health agencies, individual nursing team members, and other health professionals.

It may be determined from the case study that the infrequent visits of the client's family to her home are having a negative influence on her recovery. The nurse, as a change agent, works with the family in identifying factors influencing infrequency of visits. It may be determined that there are alterations in family processes related to fear of caring for an ill family member. Based on this nursing di-

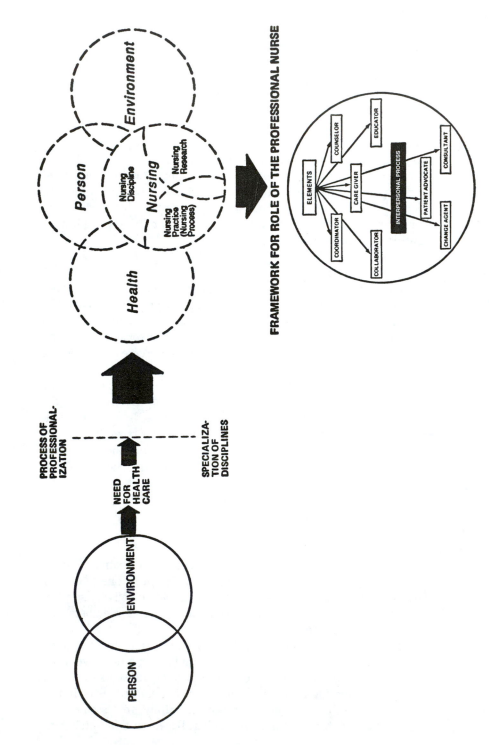

Figure 6–3. Development of the profession and discipline of nursing.

agnosis, a plan of action may be implemented to effect change in the family visiting pattern or help family members express feelings and concerns.

In summary, all of these elements interrelate and are utilized in every situation. In the example, the elements were defined separately for clarification of their meaning; however, in reality, the elements frequently overlap and the distinctions among them become less clear. For example, the nurse at times during team conferences acts as coordinator of the group in determining client goals and methods of achieving these goals. While serving as a coordinator during the conference, the nurse may also act as a consultant to another member seeking information. There may be times in the discussion when the nurse intervenes on behalf of the client and acts as a client advocate.

These elements define the role of the nurse in practice. Other professionals share some of the same elements, but they do not share the same nursing perspective developed from nursing theory and research as a basis for use of the elements. For example, a minister gives care based on theology, and a physician gives care based on medical theory and research; neither uses nursing theory or research as a basis for practice. Within nursing there are varying levels of involvement and expertise demonstrated in use of the elements because of the differing educational preparation and positions of the nurse.

Intrinsic to all of the elements are two integrating processes. The nursing process discussed earlier is a systematic goal-directed process for decision making about the delivery of nursing care based on a scientific foundation. The second integrating process is the **interpersonal process,** discussed in Chapter 2, an integral part of all nursing activities and the basis for communication between health care personnel and individuals and nurse–client–family interactions.

Figure 6–3 shows nursing with its components of discipline (theory), practice, and research arising from the foundational concepts of person, environment, and health. This forms the framework for the role of the professional nurse. The role of the professional nurse with its eight elements is illustrated with the interpersonal process as the integrating component.

THE DELIVERY OF NURSING CARE

Nurses have opportunities to provide health care in a variety of settings. Before considering these opportunities, it is valuable to look at educational preparation of nurses and numbers of nurse graduates with various educational preparation in the health care system.

Nurses are educated in college programs leading to degrees (ADN, BSN, ND, MSN, DNSc, PhD) or hospital settings (diploma) to provide client care. The elements of the role are carried out in varying degrees, depending on educational preparation and experience. For example, nurses with baccalaureate degrees in nursing have the basic skills to care for clients in a variety of settings, while nurses with master's preparation have more advanced skills. Collaborative, consultative, and coordinating skills are more highly developed with master's education. In addition, a new graduate is often less prepared to utilize the coordinator element than a registered nurse with more experience in providing client care.

 The number of nurses graduating yearly is gradually increasing, and more nurses are graduating with BSN and ADN degrees than with diplomas. For example, in 1993 there were 88,149 graduates of basic registered nurse programs. Of these, there were 24,442 baccalaureate graduates, 56,700 associate degree graduates, and 6,937 diploma graduates (National League for Nursing [NLN], 1995). Nurses prepared at master's and doctor's levels are in positions that include responsibilities of direct patient care such as nurse practitioners, nurse midwives, or nurse anesthetists or they may be in positions beyond direct patient care, such as that of a clinical nurse specialist, nurse educator, nurse researcher, or nurse administrator. The numbers of nurses prepared at these levels are increasing. In 1974, there were 2643 graduates from master's programs, whereas in 1993 there were 7926 graduates at this level. Of the total graduating with a master's degree in 1993, 755 (9.5 percent) nurses were prepared in nursing education, 1444 (18.2 percent) were prepared in nursing administration, 3429 (43.4 percent) were prepared in advanced clinical practice, 1993 (25.1 percent) prepared as nurse practitioners, and 305 (3.8 percent) in other areas (NLN, 1995). Titles for specialist positions vary within each setting; however, there are general guidelines to determine the functions of each position. Graduations of registered nurses from doctoral programs located in nursing education departments in 1974 numbered 46, compared to 381 in 1993 (NLN, 1995).

The hospital became the predominate setting for nursing practice after World War II as a result of the expansion of hospitals. Today, hospitals continue to employ the largest number of nurses, about 66.5 percent. This number continues to be relatively constant, even though nurses who are employed in hospitals may not be working in inpatient-bed units. As inpatient hospital bed occupancy continues to decline, nurses are finding employment in other areas of the hospital such as outpatient departments, operating rooms, post-anesthesia recovery units (U.S. Dept. of Health and Human Services [USDHHS], 1992). The next largest area of employment for nurses is public or community health, which also includes occupational health and school health. This area showed an increase in the early 1990s. The percentage of nurses in nursing homes and other areas of employment such as private duty and nursing education remained relatively constant during the same period (USDHHS, 1992). Figure 6–4 illustrates the estimated percentage of nurses in practice areas.

In the next section, registered nurses are discussed in terms of the approaches to the delivery of care and the elements of their role in providing primary, secondary, and tertiary care within selected health care settings. Although nurses utilize all elements of the role, only selected elements are considered for each position in the setting presented.

Types of Care Provided by Nurses

There have been various approaches to the delivery of nursing care aimed at identifying and meeting client needs within the health care delivery system. These approaches include case management; functional, team, and primary nursing approaches.

Case Management

Case management is a system with a focus on achievement of patient outcomes within a realistic time frame while being cost-effective. Case management focuses on the client for the entire episode of care and crosses all health care settings, thus simplifying the transition from one area to another. Within the case management system, a case manager, usually a nurse, maintains a caseload of clients and is responsible for developing patient outcomes. This nurse may or may not give direct client care; however, a primary

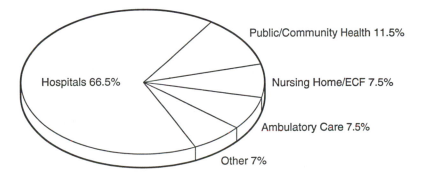

Figure 6–4. Percentage of nurses in practice areas. *(Adapted from U.S. Department of Health & Human Services. The Registered Nurse Population: Findings from the National Sample of Registered Nurses, March, 1992).*

nurse is frequently assigned by the case manager to care for particular clients. The case manager also collaborates with all health care team members to determine desirable outcomes so that a client achieves health care goals within an appropriate time frame. This type of management improves collaborative practice with all members of the health care team, decreases fragmentation, controls costs, and increases autonomy of nursing staff.

Functional Approach

The functional approach relates to the organization and distribution of tasks to facilitate efficiency of time and energy. This approach arose in the 1920s and 1930s, when American society was developing the assembly-line type of labor division. The emphasis was on maximum production at minimal cost. In nursing, this functional approach led to individuals having responsibility for a particular task, such as taking temperatures for all clients on a unit. This approach focuses on efficiency but contributes to fragmentation of care because of the emphasis on tasks rather than the client as a whole.

Team Approach

In the team approach, a nurse directs a group of persons with diversified preparation in the nursing care of clients. The nursing team traditionally involves registered nurses (RNs), licensed practical nurses (LPNs), and **unlicensed assistive personnel (UAP)** (aides, orderlies, assistants, and technicians). The nursing team combines its observations and impressions about the client, family, and significant others and the influence of the environment to provide comprehensive nursing care and guidance for caregiving. Written care plans for each client and team conferences are essential for coordination of care in the team approach. This approach gained popularity in the 1960s and aspects of the approach remain dominant today.

Primary Nursing

In primary nursing, a nurse has total responsibility for nursing care of a particular client. It differs from other methods in that responsibility for client care is assumed by the primary nurse over a 24-hour period in order to facilitate continuity of care. During the absence of the primary nurse, a secondary nurse carries out the plan of client care developed by the primary nurse, the client, and the family. There are many modifications of the primary nursing approach in use today. Primary nursing is not to be confused with primary care, which refers to health care delivery aimed at disease prevention and promotion of health. Primary care is discussed in Chapter 5.

Other Approaches

Other approaches to nursing care gaining popularity are the all-RN staff, where only registered nurses staff the unit, and independent practice, where the nurse, client, or institution mutually contract for health care.

The nursing approach used determines the way in which the nursing team is organized and influences the way nurses carry out their role. Regardless of the approach used, the nursing team includes those members involved in the nursing care of clients, their families, and significant others. The numbers and types of persons involved in nursing care are related to many factors, including the availability of nurses, philosophy of client care (e.g., beliefs about the person, rights to health care, continuity of care), and the complexity of decision making regarding nursing care needs. For example, complex decision making is often required for nursing care of acutely ill patients; thus, there is a trend away from using LPNs and auxiliary personnel to provide direct care for these clients. Increased educational preparation is being required as the basis for decision making, thereby decreasing the number of auxiliary personnel and increasing the educational preparation of nurses.

NURSING IN SELECTED PRACTICE SETTINGS

Nursing in Primary Care Settings

As described in Chapter 5, primary care is the initial health care for general complaints. It is usually the person's first contact with the health care delivery system. Primary health care providers function as a gatekeeper, managing current health care needs, preventing future problems, and referring clients to other providers and specialists when appropriate. Typical primary care services include health assessments, screening and preventive services such as blood pressure screening, nutrition counseling, immunizations, assessing and evaluating common symptoms of acute illnesses such as colds, infections, and managing chronic health problems, such as diabetes or hypertension. This care is usually provided in community settings. Even though hospitals employ over 60 percent of the registered nurses in practice, increasing numbers of nurses are being employed in community settings. The recent attention to the skyrocketing cost of hospital stays and the methods of cost containment have given impetus to alternative methods to maintain health and prevent disease at more reasonable costs.

The development of nursing's focus on community health began with Lillian Wald in 1893. Wald founded the Nurses' Settlement, which later became known as the Henry Street Settlement. The purpose of this settlement was to improve the living and health conditions of the neighborhood. The settlement was a forerunner of today's community health centers Nursing care at this time was closely aligned with Florence Nightingale's belief that improving sanitation and nutrition would promote health.

Nurses working in community settings implement many role elements in the promotion of health, one of which is educator. Community health nurses work to educate the public concerning the effects of lifestyle on health. For example, smoking and high-fat diets may contribute to heart disease.

Since the control of communicable diseases at the turn of the century, people are living longer. However, the increase in life expectancy has made the individual more prone, or susceptible, to the chronic illnesses of aging, such as heart disease, cancer, stroke, and neurological problems. Other contributors to chronic illness in America are societal influences such as stress, environmental pollutants, and substance abuse. Chronic illnesses do not necessitate hospitalization except for initial treatment and periodic therapy during exacerbations. The focus of the treatment is prevention, rehabilitation, and maintenance. This care is based in community health care settings.

Nurses provide care in community health care agencies, occupational health care agencies, rural agencies, clinics, ambulatory centers, prenatal and birthing centers, well-child centers, schools, office settings, private practice settings, private duty settings, camps, and community mental health centers.

Community Health Agencies

Community health agencies are settings where nurses implement various aspects of their role. The nurse from the community health agency may visit a client's home to identify health concerns of the client and family and to improve their understanding of health problems and health-promoting behaviors. The more familiar community agency providing this type of care is the public health agency, which is a part of the local health department and is tax-supported.

Another type of agency is the **visiting nurse association,** which is privately owned and funded by personal insurance, Medicare, Medicaid, United Way, and personal payment. Client needs may vary from primarily social to complex personal care needs. Nurses in community health agencies may be in a caregiver role to maximize personal care practices for the client and family. Family and environmental influences (such as economic and financial concerns, home safety, coping patterns, and sanitation) are major areas of concern to the nurse in this setting.

Meeting educational needs of the client is a major goal of community health nurses. For example, community health nurses may teach diabetic care; hygienic care; stress management; personal care; or skills such as changing bandages, cleaning wounds, or irrigating a colostomy. The family as well as the individual client is the focus of nursing care. The community health nurse serves as a contact person within the health care delivery system and consults and collaborates with other health care providers to meet clients' needs.

The caseload for many community health nurses varies with the location and population of clients served. Many clients are elderly and suffer from chronic illnesses. Nurses in community health settings periodically visit these clients and monitor their health status. Nurses employed in the community must be flexible and able to work independently, make health assessments, and develop plans of care for identified or potential problems. Most community health agencies require a baccalaureate degree in nursing with clinical experience in caring for adults and families. Figure 6–5 shows the nurse working in a community setting.

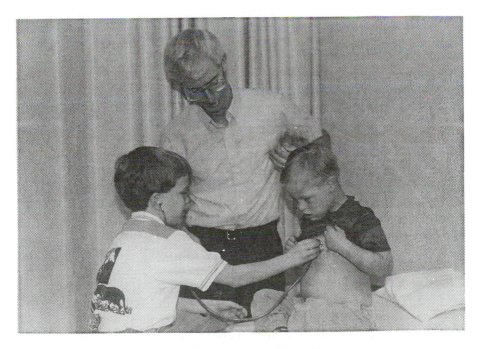

Figure 6–5. Community health nurse working with children.

Home Health Care Agencies

Home health care nursing is rapidly growing. Home health care usually refers to services and procedures provided to clients by nurses and other providers in their homes to meet actual health care needs or address potential needs. Earlier discharge of patients from hospitals, increasing number of elderly patients, cancer patients, and people with chronic illnesses who are remaining at home rather than being hospitalized are contributing to the increased need for home health services. Changes in third-party reimbursement for home services, as well as the availability of technical support that facilitates procedures such as chemotherapy, ventilators, and intravenous therapy at home, also have changed the nature of home health care.

Several types of home health care agencies are in operation today. Hospitals seeking new ways to provide service yet maintain costs have implemented home health care services as part of integrated health systems. Proprietary (for profit) agencies including insurance and pharmaceutical companies are now offering home care services as well (Spradley, 1990).

Home health care provides a broad area for the implementation of the elements of the role for nurses. Case management is typically used to organize and manage care. Needs of the clients can range from health teaching to high technological support to collaboration and consultation with other health care providers. Nurses use the various elements of the role to address the different needs of the clients.

Nursing in Occupational Health Settings

Nurses employed in occupational health settings were traditionally referred to as industrial nurses. This term developed to describe nurses who were employed by many large industries and businesses, such as the automobile and steel industries. These nurses were employed to provide basic health care and emergency treatment for employees. Since the passage of the Occupational Safety and Health Act (OSHA) in 1970, more emphasis has been placed on improving employee health as well as working conditions. It was around this time that the focus of industrial nursing widened to encompass broader health care needs of clients in an occupational setting. It has long been recognized that good employee health and working conditions can make a difference in the profitability of a company, so it is advantageous for businesses to enhance their employees' health. The focus of nurses in this setting is on caregiving and counseling. Caregiving includes screening programs for health-related problems such as diabetes mellitus, hypertension, hearing and vision impairments, and emergency care to accident victims. Counseling programs are related to health problems predominant in business and industry, such as stress management, obesity, and substance abuse.

"Occupational health nursing is the specialty practice that provides for and delivers health care services to workers and worker populations. The practice focuses on promotion, protection, and restoration of workers' health within the context of a safe and healthy work environment. Occupational health nursing practice is autonomous, and occupational health nurses make independent nursing judgments in providing occupational health services" (American Association of Occupational Health Nurses [AAOHN], 1994).

Nurses serve as consultants for business and the community in helping to establish regulations and safety programs conducive to environments that promote health. As a primary care function, the major emphasis of occupational health is on health maintenance and promotion in the workplace. Occupational health nurses are organized in the American Association of Occupational Health Nurses (AAOHN).

Working conditions for the nurse vary with the industry, and many of the nurse's fringe benefits are the same as for other employees in the industry. The job requires independence and flexibility as well as being able to interact with a variety people. The challenges of this area of community health are in health care promotion and handling of emergency situations.

Rural Nursing

Rural nursing involves health care for families who live in the rural areas and are isolated from health care facilities. These nurses visit families and make health assessments and offer emergency care, maternity care, or many other health-related interventions. Job qualifications and scope of practice vary in each state. The Frontier Nurses' Association is an example of an organization of nurses whose focus is on rural health care.

Clinics

Some clinics follow the organizational structure of the hospital with which they are affiliated. Other clinics are organized independently. Within both structures, nurses primarily utilize the elements of client educator, change agent, caregiver, and health counselor. The principal focus or goal of this type of nursing care is to assist clients in promoting and maintaining health within their home environment and social situation. Ambulatory clients with a variety of health problems (such as heart disease, chemical abuse, musculoskeletal disorders, and sensory disorders) are seen on a short-term basis. In clinics, nurses have a shorter time within each visit in which to identify these problems and assist the client in meeting the identified needs, in comparison to long-term care settings. However, since clients return to clinics in follow-up visits, nurses are able to reinforce previous teaching and to develop alternative interventions to meet the client's health care needs.

Ambulatory Care Centers

Nurses employed in ambulatory care centers provide health and follow-up care to clients who do not need overnight care. Nurses, for example, may provide pre- and postoperative teaching and care for clients undergoing same-day surgery. There is an emphasis on education for health promotion. Advanced practice nurses play important roles in providing health services in these centers.

In prenatal centers, emphasis is on teaching techniques to facilitate the labor and delivery process (such as Lamaze childbirth classes). Nurse midwives frequently practice in these centers. As the individual and family experience developmental changes, the nurse acts as a change agent in assisting them to adapt to identified needs concerning this growth. For example, a couple may attend prenatal classes taught by nurses and learn about breathing and positioning techniques to be used during the labor and delivery process. The nurse also assists the couple in learning how to provide mutual emotional support that will be needed during the birthing process and after delivery.

Prenatal and Birthing Centers

Nurses in prenatal centers primarily use the elements of caregiver, counselor, educator, and change agent to assist in the maintenance of health of the family. The nurse administers various screening procedures to identify potential health concerns. Therapeutic interpersonal skills are essential, because of the brief client contact time. Clients often need counseling regarding attitudes and beliefs about child birth and rearing, child and family development, and family relationships. Clients seen are those who need assistance in learning new, healthy lifestyles and reinforcement of existing health-promoting practices. Some areas of concern in regard to learning needs of clients may be nutrition, exercise, environmental safety, and expectations for the birthing process.

In addition to nursing in prenatal centers, nurses may care for women before, during, and after delivery in a birthing center. Nurses with advanced nursing education as midwives may assist the parents in uncomplicated deliveries. These centers have been developed to make childbirth as homelike as possible. Quite often the entire family is encouraged to participate in the birthing process.

Well-Child Centers

Care to the family following the birth of a child is also provided in well-child centers. In these centers, a new family will be guided in developmental principles of early childhood years, changes in feeding and eating habits, schedules for immunizations, and developmental milestones (crawling, standing, vocalizing, wailing, grasping, and reaching). The nurse assesses family function as well as the specific physical and emotional development of the child through screening procedures. Education, counseling regarding expectations for child behavior, and securing a safe environment are included in the nursing role. Care is provided for children in well-child centers until school age. Pediatric nurse practitioners frequently manage health care of children in well-child centers. Figure 6–6 shows the nurse conducting a teaching session with a family who has a child with Down's syndrome.

Schools

Within established educational systems, the nurse may function as an educator in health classes, a counselor for children with social or behavioral problems, a referral person for students requiring further and ongoing counseling, and a consultant for others on topics such as substance abuse, diet, nutrition, and sexuality. Disease detection, vi-

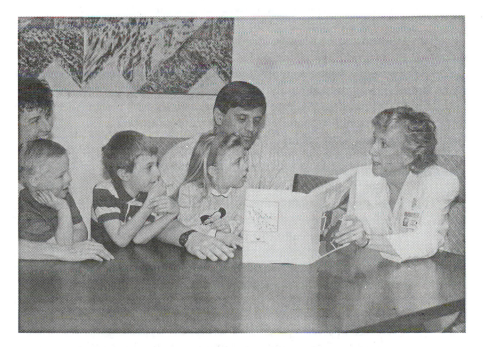

Figure 6–6. Nurse teaching a family with a child who has Down's syndrome.

sion and hearing screening, health examinations, emergency care, and environmental health and safety are important functions of the nurses in these areas. A school nurse must be able to relate to and communicate with children and be prepared to work with students with special needs. Under the Individuals with Disabilities Education Act (IDEA), students ranging from birth to adult with complex chronic physical or emotional disorders or those dependent on technology are entitled to a public education. School nurses function under the National Association of School Nurses standards of practice.

Most school systems require nurses to have a baccalaureate degree in nursing, and some school districts require nurses to be certified as school nurses or have a master's degree. Some states may also require a teaching certificate for school nurses. The application of growth and development theory, first aid skills, screening and assessment procedures, and implementation of immunization programs are common functions of the nurse in this setting. Nurses work closely with the school staff to incorporate health concepts into the curriculum and address specific child health problems.

Nursing in Office Settings

Nurses collaborate with physicians, physical therapists, and other health professionals in providing health care to clients in office settings. Depending on educational preparation, office nurses perform health assessments and provide client education. They also carry out treatments such as immunizations, dressing changes, and administration of medication. The change agent element of the nurse's role is evident in working with families and individuals to promote health-seeking behaviors and adjustments to altered family life resulting from illness of family members. Clients and families seen in office settings are often experiencing anxiety, for which the nurse provides emotional support and comfort. Educational requirements vary, as do the hours of employment.

Nursing in Private Practice Settings

Private practice indicates that nurses, usually advanced practice nurses, individually or as a group, practice nursing in self-employed settings. This type of practice provides the public with an alternative in the type of health care provider, allows the nurse to establish direct client contact revolving around identified nursing care needs, facilitates continuity of nursing care, and provides accountability for nursing through direct fee for services.

Areas for private practice in nursing today include psychiatric mental health, adult and family, and community health practice. Nurses in private practice, as in all other types of practice, utilize interpersonal skills and the nursing process to identify, meet, and evaluate client needs. All elements of the role are applied in order to promote health.

Private Duty Nursing

Private duty nursing may be referred to as the forerunner of private practice. Nurses are contracted by individual clients, families, or home health agencies to provide one-to-one care within a variety of settings (hospitals, homes, extended care facilities). Private duty nurses frequently gain satisfaction from the direct and personal contact with clients. Requests for private duty nurses are increasing as more patients leave the hospital sooner and are in need of nursing care at home. Nurses in private duty and working in a health care facility must practice in accord with the policies of the facility in which they are working.

Within the home, the nurse works within the expectations of the family and the limitations of the home setting. Elements of the role are implemented to various degrees, depending on the setting and client needs.

Camp Nursing

Camp nursing can provide an alternative to the usual areas of nursing employment. Nurses in a camp situation usually work independently. They provide for preventive and acute health care needs. In camps that specialize in children with certain health problems, such as diabetes mellitus, obesity, or various physical challenges, the nurse assists the campers with their special health care needs.

Camp nurses are actively involved with the development and implementation of health programs for campers, their families, and the camp staff and with the administration of first aid for injuries, treatments, and medications. Camp nurses must have cardiopulmonary resuscitation (CPR) certification as well as first-aid training. Experience in emergency, community health, and pediatric nursing can be an asset. Camp nursing jobs are usually seasonal (i.e., for a specific span of time such as the summer) and the hours are often long, with modest financial reimbursement. Some camps do have provisions for the family of the camp nurse. Persons who enjoy the outdoors usually find camp nursing to be challenging. Employment qualifications vary with the size of the camp, health status of the campers, job responsibilities, state and local health codes, and any specific criteria defined by the camp.

Community Mental Health Agencies

Community mental health agency services assist clients to maintain their functioning within society while receiving treatment. The nurse acts as a counselor to the client and as a consultant to other health professionals. Nurses also assist significant others in health promotion activities of the client. The emphasis of the caregiver element is on psychological care and emotional support. Nurses assess patterns of interaction and the effects of the interaction on the clients' functioning within the family or the community. In the situation where the family is the client, assessment is made of individual patterns of interaction within the family and of family functioning within the community. Numerous therapeutic approaches may be employed to meet the clients' psychological needs. Advanced educational preparation in nursing is required for the nursing position in most community mental health agencies.

Nursing in Correctional Facilities

Prisoners in correctional facilities have health care needs the same as the general population. They may be in need of emergency care or have chronic illnesses such as hypertension, diabetes, heart disease, cancer; or problems with substance abuse; or pregnancy. Inmates with acute problems are generally transferred to local hospitals, but health education and promotion are important aspects of the role of the nurse. Other areas for nursing intervention, such as first aid, health assessments, screening for infectious diseases (especially HIV and hepatitis B), and mental health care are within the realm of nursing.

Nursing in the Military

Nursing in the military can provide many opportunities including travel both in the United States and abroad, education reimbursement for advanced study, officer rank for those with BSN degrees, and opportunity to work in specialty hospitals. Military nurses often have many options for service including active or reserve duty or a combination. Retirement benefits are also very appealing for nurses making a military career.

Nursing Entrepreneurs

The changes in third-party payment in the past few years enabling nurses to receive payment for services has increased the interest in advanced practice nurses establishing themselves in private or joint practice with other health care professionals. Knowledge of the particular state board regulations governing nursing practice is essential, as well as ability to secure third-party reimbursement. Nurses in private practice often find business and management skills are essential to organize and implement the practice.

Nursing in Secondary Care Settings

As stated in Chapter 5, hospitals are the major facilities for provision of secondary health care. Hospitals also employ the largest percentage of registered nurses (66 percent). Nurses in these settings practice nursing in positions that require the use of the elements of the professional nurse's role. Organization within the hospital is complexly structured because of the number of services and personnel. Well-defined organizational patterns are characteristic of hospitals. Organizational models outline the communication structure within institutions and departments. Many hospitals are now part of integrated health systems.

Nursing service, one unit of the hospital, is organized according to various models. In each model there exists a nurse who has the overall responsibility for nursing services. Some titles for this position are director of nursing service, assistant or associate administrator for nursing, and vice-president for nursing.

Nurses who serve as liaisons between the director of nursing service and individual nursing units are nursing supervisors or clinical coordinators. Nurses responsible for the overall coordination of individual nursing units are head nurses and assistant head nurses. In some organizations the clinical nurse specialist is responsible for the coordination of the nursing unit. In other organizations the clinical specialist has other responsibilities. This position is discussed later in the chapter. Typically, administrative positions of nurses in hospitals include director of nursing service, supervisor or coordinator, head nurse, and sometimes clinical specialist.

Common functions of nurses in administrative positions are participation in the development and implementation of a philosophy for nursing service and in budgeting, staffing, coordinating, and decision making for designated areas of responsibility. Within the individual nursing units, staff and general duty nurses are responsible for direct nursing care. Staff or general duty positions are not administrative.

Vice-President or Director of Nursing

The entire nursing service department within the facility is the responsibility of the vice-president or director of nursing. The person in this position is accountable to the administrator of the hospital and often serves as an assistant or associate administrator. In this position, the director interprets current nursing trends to the hospital administrator, presents proposed plans for change, and seeks support for needed resources. The director must make sure that institutional priorities are not in conflict with the goals, standards, and priorities of the nursing profession. In consultation with the supervisors and head nurses, the director of nursing assesses nursing services, establishes long- and short-term goals consistent with the philosophy of the institution, implements plans to meet the goals, and evaluates the process and outcomes of the plans. The director of nursing is responsible for initiating and maintaining structures for developing and implementing nursing standards, policies, and procedures.

Clinical Coordinator

Clinical coordinators are middle managers who have administrative responsibility for more than one patient care or specialty unit such as orthopedics, oncology, surgery, or medicine. They are in charge of the administrative functions for large groups of clients and several patient care areas. Clinical coordinators make overall observations concerning client care and unit functioning and provide direction in terms of proposed changes, developmental programs, and staff education. Coordinators also assist in establishment and implementation of policies. In this position, the nurse must be thoroughly knowledgeable about the overall organization, functioning, policies, and procedures of the hospital. Major elements of the role of these positions include consultation and collaboration as well as coordination. Persons in such a position should be aware of new trends and research in nursing and be able to convey this information to others. As liaison between the director of nursing and the head nurse, the coordinator must be skilled in the interpersonal process. There are usually several clinical coordinators in a hospital. One of the clinical coordinators may act as the assistant director of nursing service.

Unit Manager or Head Nurse

The major responsibility of the unit manager or head nurse is coordination of care on individual patient care units. To reflect the administrative role of the head nurse, many institutions have changed the title of head nurse to unit manager.

In collaboration with staff nurses, the unit manager assigns nursing care responsibilities to team members and has the overall responsibility for ensuring that the nursing care is planned and implemented for each assessed need.

Orientation, professional development, evaluation, and guidance of nursing personnel is another administrative function of this position. The unit manager generally assumes responsibility for client nursing care on a 24-hour basis and serves as a role model for personnel. The unit manager also coordinates nonnursing personnel who provide the support services such as clerical work, equipment and supply acquisition, and other nonnursing aspects of the unit.

Staffing and budgeting of individual units may or may not be the responsibility of the unit manager. In some organizations the clinical specialist assumes the unit manager title, but there are different job expectations.

Staff Nurse

Probably the most common nursing position in the hospital is related to direct client care. Nurses in this position are most often referred to as general duty or staff nurses. In general, the staff nurse does not become directly involved in the administrative management of the unit. Some typical functions of the staff nurse are assessment of patient health care needs and planning and implementing interventions; promotion of psychological support for clients, family, and significant others (such as assisting in maintaining health patterns for stress reduction and verbalizing concerns, feelings, and fears); performance of psychomotor skills (such as range-of-motion exercises, maintenance of fluid balance via intravenous therapy, provision of comfort measures, changing dressings, and administering medication); and evaluation of care.

The staff nurse, as client advocate, is spokesperson for ensurance of client's rights by other health care providers and significant others. This element has particular importance today because of the tendency toward fragmented care resulting from the client's contact with a large number of health care providers. The nurse as client advocate intervenes to ensure that all identified needs of the client are considered. The staff nurse is usually the first to become aware of areas the client is dissatisfied with or expresses concern regarding hospitalization. The resolution of these concerns with other health providers and services within the hospital is part of the function of the staff nurse as a coordinator of care. Figure 6–7 shows a nurse conducting play therapy with children in a pediatric setting. Figure 6–8 shows a nursing instructor teaching a nursing student to use equipment for client care.

Coordination also involves communication with other nursing team members regarding identification of needs and plans to meet these needs through written care plans and nursing team conferences. The staff nurse continually acts as an educator to clients and other nursing team members. Common educational topics for client needs include treatments, transfer techniques, medications, community services, postoperative care, disease processes, self-care, and health-promoting behaviors. The framework for decision making concerning nursing actions is the nursing process, which is based on theory and research. Communication through the interpersonal process is essential in utilization of all elements of the role.

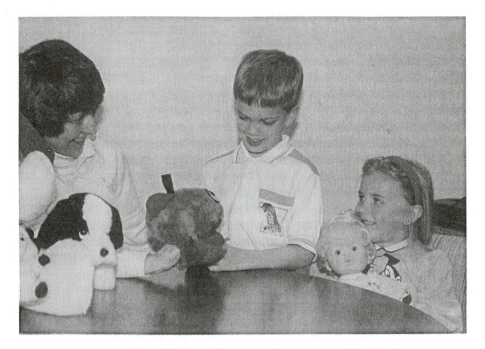

Figure 6–7. Play therapy with children.

An example of how nurses in various positions work together for the improvement of client care follows.

> An existing policy provides that parents may visit toddlers on pediatric units only during established visiting hours. Staff nurses consistently observe that toddlers are experiencing anxiety when separated from their parents. This problem is conveyed to the head nurse. After consultation, the unit manager may determine that, taking into account observations and studies indicating the negative effects of separation for this age child, the policy should be reviewed and discussed with the director of nursing. It may be decided that, for an experimental period, an alternative visiting policy should be implemented and evaluated. The vice-president of nursing would then present the proposal through the appropriate channels for policy change. Any resulting policy change would be communicated to appropriate department personnel.

The way in which patient care units are organized within the hospital depends on the organizational structure, size and focus of the hospital, and the needs of the community. This also applies to divisions within specialty hospitals. For example, pediatric hospitals may have units based on age groups, medical classifications of disease processes, or acuteness of patient illness. The most common

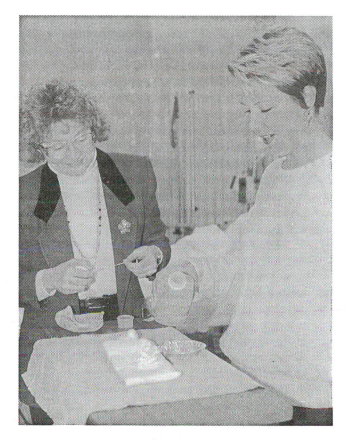

Figure 6–8. Nursing student in the hospital.

method of organizing units is according to medically determined client care classifications (e.g., pediatric, obstetric, medical, surgical, psychiatric, or orthopedic). Nurses in each of these types of units utilize the role elements based on theory related to the area of specialization. For example, on a pediatric unit, nurses work with children of all ages. Their role is based on theory related to growth and developmental principles, effects of hospitalization and treatment methods on children, and the effects of illness and specific child-related disease processes on the child and family. On an obstetric unit, nurses are in contact with families during the three stages of pregnancy; prenatal (prior to birth), intrapartal (during the birth process), and postpartal (after the birth process). Employing the nursing process, the nurse gives care focusing on safe labor and delivery and the adjustment of the family to the change in family structure.

Other types of units are the specialized care units. These units may be classified as coronary care, medical intensive care, surgical intensive care, neurological intensive care, burn intensive care, operating room, labor and delivery, oncology, trauma, postanesthesia care, or psychiatric care. Clients are admitted to these units for intensive nursing and medical care. Physical care and emotional support of clients and significant others in time of crisis are essential. Nursing in specialized care units is based on theory related to areas such as crisis, stress, and physiological processes.

The emergency department is another specialized unit. In this unit, nurses rapidly assess and make decisions related to specific traumas such as accidents, burns, strokes, and heart attacks. Interpersonal skills are crucial because of the high stress level of clients and families in these crisis situations.

Life flight is a recent concept that extends emergency nursing and medical care into the community. The life flight involves a helicopter and health care team that includes a pilot and health care professionals, who may include a nurse and physician. Life flight was developed to meet the needs of people not readily accessible to health care by normal vehicles or where quick transportation to a trauma center is necessary. During the flight from the accident area to the hospital, the victim is monitored and life supports are initiated as necessary. Nurses employed as life flight nurses usually have extensive experiences in emergency care. Those who enjoy the challenges of emergency care may find nursing in life flight an alternative to nursing in emergency settings. This type of service is available only in selected health care settings.

Nurses provide care to persons admitted to units specializing in general medical-surgical care. Clients may be admitted directly or by transfer from more acute settings such as intensive care units. In addition to initiating and providing care, home-going instruction and discharge planning is implemented for the client and family. Personal care and involvement of family in the client's care are stressed.

In addition to the nursing positions discussed, there is another nursing position supportive to client care. This is the position of the infection surveillance nurse, who establishes programs and policies for infection control and coordinates and educates hospital personnel to recognize and report communicable disease. Recognition of the presence of infectious processes contributes to the identification of causative agents and methods to control further transmission of infection. The primary emphasis of the nurse in this position is on preventing the incidence of hospital-acquired (nosocomial) infection.

Another position is that of nurse educator. The educator element is part of each nurse's role; however, positions have developed within nursing that are particularly supportive of this element. Some nurse leaders advocate master's preparation in nursing for specialized nurse educator positions; however, this has not been realized in many clinical settings. Therefore, we include the role in this section rather than in the section on nursing specialists. One type of nurse educator position is that of the client educator. The client educator position is specifically designed to help staff nurses meet the teaching needs of clients. In some institutions, the client educator works primarily with the staff in facilitating the planning and implementing of teaching plans. In other settings, the educator plans and implements the teaching plan directly with clients and families, and maintains communication with the staff concerning the teaching. In both instances, the client educator is a consultant for client education problems.

In addition to working at the individual client level, the nurse in this position is responsible for identifying client education needs on a broader scale and coordinating efforts to develop teaching programs. For example, a client educator may develop a plan for teaching clients before and after surgery. The plan may include specific content to be taught, methods for teaching (booklets, slides, etc.), and rationale for the content. This plan may be carried out by the client educator with reinforcement from the staff or by the staff nurse with the client in a one-to-one interaction. Client educators may be employed in the generalized area of client education or in specialized areas. Some specialized areas of client education include diabetic teaching, ostomy teaching (colostomy or ileostomy), cardiac instruction, IV therapy, and weight control.

Another type of nurse educator position is that of staff development. Nurses in staff development have two major areas of responsibility. The first area of responsibility is to plan, provide, and evaluate orientation programs for personnel new to the facility. The purpose of the orientation program is to familiarize new nurse employees with the philosophy, policies, and procedures of the institution, and to serve as a resource guide during the new employee's period of adjustment. The second area is to identify learning needs among nursing personnel in the facility or organization. The nurse in staff development institutes in-service programs for reviewing skills and presenting new equipment, procedures, and policies. The focus of the educational program is on professional development of individuals within their role. Coordination of continuing education is a related area that involves conducting continuing education programs within the institution and arranging for staff attendance at programs outside the facility.

Nursing in Tertiary Prevention Care Settings

Clients needing long-term and rehabilitation services receive those services in tertiary prevention care settings. Nursing in long-term care consists of providing nursing care, skilled care, and rehabilitation for all age groups. Long-term care is more than just caring for the small portion (about 5 percent) of the aging population needing to be institutionalized in a formal setting such as a nursing home. It is providing long-term care to anyone with health care needs amenable to nursing intervention. Children as well as adults with debilitating chronic illnesses often need long-term care. This care can take place in many settings such as the person's home, in group homes, or in specific facilities or institutions for long-term care. Long-term care can be a challenging area of practice especially for nurses who like to care for clients over a long period of time.

Nursing in Skilled Care Settings

Skilled care facilities are long-term care settings for geriatric clients and others requiring continued care, such as clients with brain injury and neurological impairments. These facilities include residential accommodations for ambulatory, self-care clients as well as nursing care units for patients requiring varying degrees of nursing care. In addition, some of these facilities provide day centers where the elderly may come for group or social interaction. Nursing care is designed and delivered on the basis of theory related to gerontology and includes assessing needs and providing and evaluating care through the use of the nursing process and expressed through the elements of the nurse's role. The structure of nursing positions within these settings is similar to those in hospitals and includes director of nursing, supervisor or clinical coordinator, head nurse, and staff nurse. There is impetus from societal and governmental groups to increase the number of professional nursing personnel within these facilities. As a caregiver within these facilities, the nurse provides nursing care for clients with chronic or long-term illness. The emphasis is on promoting and maintaining personal care in activities of daily living or enhancing the optimum level of functioning. Nurses as caregivers assist the elderly in adjusting to the physical and psychosocial changes of aging.

The elderly experience changes in social structure related to several areas. One of these is the movement in American society away from the extended family toward a nuclear family structure. Another change for the elderly is the loss of significant others through death. With changing family and social structure, there may not be significant others available to support the elderly in decision making. Often the nurse must assume this responsibility by ensuring that adequate services are provided and that dignity is maintained. Integral to the loss of significant others is the awareness on the part of the elderly of their own impending death. Nurses must support the client in working through these feelings and assist them in coping with their losses. Nurses as patient advocates are primary change agents in affecting positive societal attitudes toward the elderly.

Nursing in Rehabilitation Settings

Clients are usually admitted to rehabilitation facilities following an acute illness resulting in some type of impairment that interferes with individual care and maintenance of health. Children may also be admitted to rehabilitation facilities due to developmental delays resulting at birth or from trauma. Rehabilitation involves the client and others in care measures aimed at restoring the person's health to its maximum potential (often within the confines of a chronic disease process or physical or developmental change). There is an increased emphasis on the interdisciplinary health care team as the primary provider of health services in this setting. Rehabilitation facilities and nursing staff are organized in much the same way as hospitals and skilled care facilities.

Nursing in a rehabilitation setting, as in other settings, is based on a holistic approach to client care, focusing on the physical, psychosocial, and spiritual aspects of the person. Some major areas of emphasis for care giving in rehabilitation are the prevention of complications such as pressure ulcers (bedsores) and muscle contractures, provision of comfort measures, and psychological support. Nurses, in collaboration with other health professionals, spend a majority of their time working as change agents and educators in assisting clients to relearn previously acquired skills, to learn new health-promoting skills related to the activities of daily living, and new behaviors to compensate for physical changes. For example, a nurse may identify teaching needs in the areas of exercise, transfer techniques, bowel and bladder training, and weight control for a client who is paraplegic (with paralysis of the lower extremities).

The interplay of the elements of caregiver, counselor, and educator is evident as the nurse assists the client in adjusting to the changes in body image. Psychological support is essential for clients in rehabilitation facilities. The nurse must also assist the family and significant others with their adjustment to new roles and lifestyles, such as living with a person who has limited activity caused by respiratory impairment.

Use of the nursing process to establish a plan of care and communication of this plan is essential to rehabilitation, as in all areas of nursing. Clients in rehabilitation facilities often need the services of other health care providers such as physical, speech, and occupational therapists and psychologists with whom the nurse collaborates and consults. A function of the nurse for successful rehabilitation of clients is the coordination of the care given by all health care providers

Hospice Nursing

Hospice nursing is an old aspect of care, dating back to the Middle Ages, when tired travelers could seek food and shelter in a hospice. The modern concept of hospice is identified with St. Christopher's Hospice in London, where terminally ill persons receive health care. In the United States, hospice care has been developed to care for terminally ill clients and their families in their home. The care provided is palliative and supportive. The nurse utilizes the role element of coordinator to organize the care over a 24-hour period. Hospice care involves many volunteers and members of the health team. Health team conferences with all involved health care providers are not unusual and must be coordinated. The counselor element of the nurse's role is used to support family and client during the illness phase as well as the bereavement of the family after the client's death.

Employment in hospice care is demanding, since the care of persons who are terminally ill can be emotionally draining. Emotional stability and maturity are necessary qualifications. There are no specific educational qualifications to be a hospice nurse. Some agencies prefer nurses with a baccalaureate degree.

ADVANCED PRACTICE NURSING

Advanced practice nurses (APN) is a broad term for nurses who have completed educational preparation at the graduate level to acquire the needed knowledge and practice experiences for specialization (ANA, 1995). In the past some advanced preparation requirements were met with certificate programs beyond the RN and many of these nurses continue to practice in advanced practice roles. However, because of the complexity of clinical decision making, in-depth knowledge of theories, application of research, and specialized skills, APNs require education at the graduate level (Frik & Pollock, 1993). Nurse practitioners (NP), clinical nurse specialists (CNS), certified nurse midwives (CNM), and nurse anesthetists (CRNA) are the nurses usually considered to be practicing in advanced practice roles (National Council of State Boards of Nursing [NCSBN], 1992). At the 1992 ANA Congress of Nursing Practice the following definition of advanced practice was approved:

> Nurses in advanced clinical nursing practice have a graduate degree in nursing. They conduct comprehensive health assessments, demonstrate a high level of autonomy and possess expert skill in the diagnosis and treatment of complex responses of individual, families and communities to actual or potential health problems. They formulate clinical decisions to manage acute and chronic ill-

ness and promote wellness. Nurses in advanced practice integrate education, research, management, leadership and consultation into their clinical role and function in collegial relationships with nursing peers, physicians, professional and others who influence the health environment (ANA, 1992).

The shift in health care focus to primary care has increased the need for APNs. APNs can provide primary and preventive care with cost-effective quality (Sweet, 1986). In recent years there has been debate over whether the roles of NP and CNS should merge or continue to be separate. The two roles have similar conceptual foundations but they have developed as separate entities. Historically, the NP practiced primarily in primary care settings and the CNS usually provided care in secondary and tertiary care settings. With the shift to more health promotion and primary care, the roles in these practice settings have become less clear. The debate on whether to merge the two roles will continue (Page & Arena, 1994).

Nurse Practitioner

The NP movement has its roots at the University of Colorado, where the first NP program was developed by Ford and Silver in response to a shortage of primary care physicians in 1967. This program was designed as a postbaccalaureate program to prepare nurses for an expanded role in child care. The **nurse practitioner** movement grew as more federal funding became available in the 1970s. Many programs ranged from 4 months to 2 years and were certificate programs. The original intent was to develop graduate level programs, but societal demand for NPs led to continuing education certificate programs. Recently, movement by nursing organizations has shifted the educational focus from a certificate program to a graduate level program (Kelly, 1994; Snyder, 1995). Assessment skills are used, primarily in ambulatory settings, with a variety of clients and age groups. Assessment includes determining physical and psychosocial health status of patients through history and physical examinations, and evaluating and interpreting findings in order to plan and carry out interventions. NPs practice in many areas such as pediatrics, family health, adult, geriatrics, community health, and mental health. More recently, there has been a demand for NPs in acute-care settings. Currently there are separate certification examinations for primary care and acute-care NPs. (See Figure 6–9.)

Clinical Nurse Specialist

CNSs have master's degrees in a clinical specialty area (e.g., adult nursing, psychiatric and mental health nursing, maternal–child nursing, psychosocial nursing, emergency nursing, and geriat-

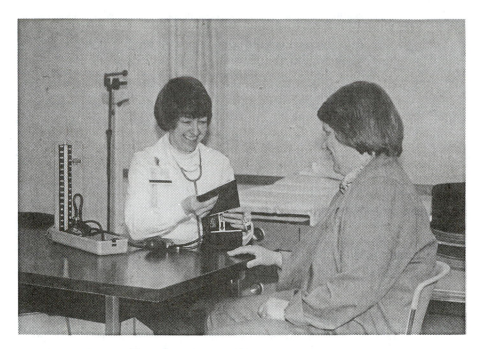

Figure 6–9. Nurse conducting a health assessment.

ric nursing). With this additional nursing education, CNSs are able to provide advanced levels of client care and assist other health professionals in establishing and meeting health goals. The educational preparation places emphasis on collaboration and consultation with other health care providers who may need help dealing with complex client problems. Traditionally, CNSs have focused on specific groups of clients with common problems, for example, adult clients who have been diagnosed with cancer. They are employed in private practice as well as health care delivery settings. Clinical specialists frequently engage in research to improve care to clients.

Certified Nurse Midwife

CNMs provide prenatal, intrapartal, and postpartal care to expectant families. They are educated in normal obstetrics and gynecology and are certified by the American College of Nurse Midwives. Advanced education, post-RN, occurs in accredited programs of varying lengths. The trend is toward requiring a master's degree for this type of practice.

CNMs conduct prenatal health examinations, manage normal labor and delivery, well-woman gynecology, and educate and counsel families in infant care, nutrition, and family planning. A license to practice is determined by the individual state, but at this time not all states have licensure regulating nurse midwife practice.

A major emphasis of the CNM role is women's health. The major part of the CNM's practice is with families where a normal pregnancy, labor, and delivery are anticipated. When a potential for complications arises, a CNM consults with a physician. The American College of Nurse Midwives (ACNM) is the professional organization for nurse midwives.

Nurse Anesthetist

Nurses who specialize in the administration of anesthesia after completing an accredited program of nurse anesthesia are referred to as *nurse anesthetists*. These nurses are then able to use the title CRNA. Schools of nurse anesthesia require applicants to have a baccalaureate degree in nursing or a related field, an RN license, and nursing experience. Program lengths vary from 18 to 27 months. Some schools award a certificate on graduation. In other schools the program is part of a master's degree program. By 1998, all programs will offer a master's degree.

Nursing Positions Requiring Higher Degree Preparation

In addition to APN, where the term refers to clinical practice, there are many other advanced positions for nurses who are educated at the master's and doctor's level, including nurse educator, nurse administrator, nurse consultant, and nurse researcher.

Nurse Educator

Education is one of nursing's oldest specialty areas and has been presented as a role element for all nurses. This section deals with the nurse who teaches within formal nursing educational settings. There were 270,228 students enrolled in basic nursing education programs in 1993 (NLN, 1995). In addition, there were 30,385 students enrolled in master's programs and 2,754 enrolled in nursing doctoral programs in the same year. The nurse educator prepares the nursing student in nursing theory, research, and practice. At the basic level, students are prepared for licensure as registered nurses. In general, the educational requirement for nurses employed in nursing education is a master's degree in nursing, with a doctorate preferred for baccalaureate and higher-degree education. Responsibilities of the nurse educator include curriculum development (such as developing philosophy, establishing goals, planning courses and teaching methods), curriculum implementation and evaluation, and development, counseling, and advising of students. Faculty members are also responsible for participating in research and other scholarly endeavors as well as providing service to the educational institution and community. They conduct and participate in continuing education programs for health professionals.

Nurse educators utilize the caregiver element by being role models for students and staff in clinical settings and by participating in direct client care. It is important that nurse educators maintain clinical competence in nursing practice. Since nurse educators function within several systems concurrently (educational system, health care delivery system, and community system), the coordinator, collaborator, and consultant elements are frequently implemented.

Nurse Administrator

Nurse administrators function in schools of nursing, health care facilities, and other professional and health-related agencies. They are accountable for ensuring that all of the professional nurses within their area of responsibility implement the elements of the nursing role. They ensure that professional goals are maintained and that an environment conducive to the discipline of nursing is provided.

Within schools of nursing, nurse administrators provide guidance for curriculum development, recruit quality nurse educators, and collaborate with other administrators in ascertaining resources for teaching and practice. They facilitate and are supportive of research, publications, and other creative works that contribute to the discipline of nursing. Nurse administrators within health care facilities coordinate nursing services within their facility and guide the philosophy, policies, and procedures within the facilities to be consistent with professional goals. The nurse administrator is professionally accountable and committed to the promotion of the discipline. Nurse administrators are responsible for contributing to ongoing research in nursing.

Nurse administrators work within health care facilities as directors of nursing service, supervisors and coordinators, or head nurses. In these positions, they are responsible for overall organization and administration of nursing services. Staffing, budgeting, and policy making are principal administrative responsibilities. In addition, nurse administrators function as liaisons with other professionals in the health care setting. Key elements used by nurse administrators are collaboration, coordination, and consultation. They implement new concepts in nursing and must be aware of current trends.

Nurses work in various administrative positions in the profession and in government. They have power and influence to effect changes for the enhancement of nursing practice. These changes may be in the form of legislation, establishment of programs for nursing and health care, or influencing decisions related to established programs and policies. For instance, there are full-time nurses working at the state level to establish and maintain state boards of nursing education and nurse registration.

Nurses are in administrative positions in local, state, and federal health coordinating agencies. Nurses administer professional and other nursing organizations such as the American Nurses Association and the National League for Nursing. Nurses also are employed in administrative positions at the international level (e.g., World Health Organization, International Council for Nurses).

Nurse Consultant

Nurse consultants can work in a variety of settings, depending on the area of expertise. Consultation can occur in any nursing setting. Consultation with school personnel is for the purpose of developing and evaluating curriculums. Private consultants respond to a particular client requests, such as improving staffing patterns in a hospital or improving the communication network. Most consultants are paid a fee for services and utilize various elements of the role extensively.

Nurse Researcher

Nurse researchers are skilled in the research process, which is aimed at improving patient care and validating theory in nursing practice. These nurses are proficient in problem solving, in assessing situations to develop research studies, and in investigating theoretical and clinical problems. Nurse researchers must be able to write clearly and succinctly in order to disseminate research findings. College schools of nursing currently employ nurse researchers. Recently, health care facilities have begun to employ nurse researchers for clinical nursing research. These nurses serve to advance the discipline of nursing through theory development and validation, thereby improving client care. The majority of nurse researchers have either master's or doctor's degrees. Further development of the nurse as researcher is presented in Chapter 7.

CLINICAL PRACTICE AS A STUDENT

Delivery of nursing care to meet actual or potential client health needs and promote health is the focus of nursing. Therefore, as part of the educational process and role development as a nurse, it is necessary to learn how theory from nursing, art, humanities, and science relates to clinical practice. This knowledge base is gained through didactic content and clinical practice in community agencies and hospitals under the supervision of nursing faculty. This section discusses the clinical practice component of the educational process as a method of implementing nursing theory and research and of demonstrating the elements of the role of the nurse. Most students are eager to start clinical experience with clients from the day they decide to enter a nursing program. Clinical experience in various health care agencies usually begins after an introduction to the arts, humanities, and sciences. Nursing services are provided by students under the supervision of the educational institution.

As a student progresses through a baccalaureate program, the clinical experience becomes more varied as the view of the client expands to include family and community members. Liberal arts courses, taken primarily during the first 2 years of study but continuing through the last years, provide the basis for this expanding view. The student becomes familiar with different hospital units and community agencies as well as with functional aspects of the nurses' role in these areas. Curriculum control is under the auspices of faculty and administration of the institution.

In the associate degree programs, students usually affiliate with local health agencies; the faculty and institutional administration govern the curriculum. The basic liberal arts courses are taken concurrently with nursing courses. The goals for clinical practice differ from those of the baccalaureate programs, as discussed in the previous section.

Most diploma programs enroll their students for basic liberal arts courses at a local college or university while they begin nursing courses within a hospital setting. Diploma programs are under the auspices of the hospital administration. Students in these programs receive most of their clinical practice in the same facility.

The student's actual clinical experience will vary with the individual school, its philosophy and available facilities. An instructor usually assigns students to provide short-term nursing care to clients. The assignments are based on student learning objectives for the day. Students may be assigned to a new client each week or care for the same one over an extended period of time. This care may be given in traditional hospital settings, in other health care agencies, or in nonstructured health care settings. In all programs the clinical practice component remains client centered.

Confidence in nursing practice is developed as the student cares for a client and works to identify and meet a variety of health care needs. The student generally prepares a plan of nursing care for meeting these needs and for evaluating care. This **nursing care plan** is developed using the nursing process and is based on principles, facts, concepts, theory, and research; it provides a process for decision making and addresses health care needs of the client.

A typical clinical day may begin with a preconference, where students share plans for the day with other members of the clinical group. Or students may join in walking rounds with other staff as a means of continuity of client care. Usually an instructor will be responsible for six to ten students in the clinical area. This ratio usually depends on the nature of the assignment and the supervision the student needs to provide safe care to the client. The major part of the clinical time will consist of actual client care with supervision from the instructor, followed by a postconference to evaluate the day's care. Seminars may be held for discussion of students' clinical experiences. Faculty supervision of students is based on teaching-learning principles, the clinical setting, and the learning needs of the students. Some type of written assignment usually is required to enhance the learning experience. Use of nursing process is stressed in clinical situations. See the discussion of nursing process earlier in this chapter.

SUMMARY

The actual implementation of theory is in the clinical or practice setting. Professional practice has a knowledge base and is guided by standards of practice. The nursing process was viewed as a deliberative, systematic approach to nursing care based on scientific inquiry and problem-solving methods. The characteristics and steps to the process were discussed. The role of the nurse has been discussed in settings within the health care delivery system. Nurses can also become involved in health care through informal means by incorporating cultural beliefs of the clients in planned nursing actions, community educational programs, and private practice.

Nurses function in various settings to meet client needs. Nurses in any of these settings continue to use the nursing process and interpersonal process as they utilize all elements of the role: caregiver, client advocate, counselor, educator, coordinator, collaborator, consultant, and change agent. All nurses work within specific practice limits and state and federal regulations in these settings. Within all of the health care settings, the nurse utilizes theoretical knowledge and research findings in carrying out the elements of the role in practice.

▶ Questions for Discussion

1. List the characteristics of the nursing process.
2. List the components of the nursing process.
3. There are several types of skills involved in nursing practice. Describe at least three.
4. Can you think of a health problem that you (or someone you know) has and apply the nursing process framework to it?

5. Choose two nursing settings and discuss similarities and differences between the nursing positions and functions within these settings.
6. How do the nurse educator and nurse administrator implement the role of the nurse?
7. Does the emphasis on specific elements of the role of the nurse change from setting to setting? For example, are the major elements for a nurse practicing in a hospital situation the same as those for a nurse practicing in a community agency?
8. How will advance practice nurses address health care needs?
9. What type of nursing program are you attending, and what is the basic curriculum design?
10. What are the clinical facilities used by your nursing program?
11. What is the philosophy of your school of nursing?

REFERENCES

Adam E. *To Be a Nurse*. 2nd ed. Philadelphia: Saunders; 1991.

American Association of Occupational Health Nurses. *Standards of Occupational Health Nursing Practice*. Atlanta, GA: AAOHN, 1994.

American Nurses Association Congress of Nursing Practice. *Working Definition: Nurses in Advanced Clinical Practice*. Washington, D.C.: ANA; 1992.

American Nurses Association. *Nursing's Social Policy Statement*. Washington D.C.: American Nurses Publishing; 1995.

American Nurses Association. *Standards of Clinical Nursing Practice*. Washington D.C.: American Nurses Publishing; 1991.

Bandman E, Bandman B. *Critical Thinking in Nursing*. 3rd ed. Norwalk, CT: Appleton & Lange; 1995.

Brooks J, Kleine-Krachl A. Evaluation of a definition of nursing. *Adv Nurs Sci* 1983; 5:61–85.

Bulechek G, McCloskey J. *Nursing Interventions: Essential Nursing Treatments*. 2nd ed. Philadelphia: Saunders; 1992.

Carpenito L. *Handbook of Nursing Diagnosis*. 6th ed. Philadelphia: Lippincott; 1995.

Carpenito L. The NANDA Definition of Nursing Diagnosis: Proceedings of the Ninth Conference. In: Carroll-Johnson, ed. *Classification of Nursing Diagnoses*. Philadelphia: JB Lippincott; 1991.

Conley M. Management effectiveness and the role making process. *Nurs Admin*. 1974; 4:6.

Frik S, Pollock S. Preparation for advanced nursing practice. *Nurs Health Care*. 1993; 14(4):190–195.

Gordon M. Nursing diagnosis and the diagnostic process. *Am J Nurs.* 1976; 76:1298–1300.

Gordon M. *Nursing Diagnosis: Process and Application.* 2nd ed. New York: McGraw-Hill; 1987.

Keller N. The why and whats of private practice. *J Nurs Admin.* 1973; 5:15.

Kelley, Jean. Looking ahead to 21st century master's nursing education. In: *A Changing Health Care System.* Southern Council on Collegiate Education for Nursing. Atlanta: 1994; 11–30.

Leddy S & Pepper JM. *Conceptual Bases of Professional Nursing.* 3rd ed. Philadelphia: JB Lippincott; 1993.

McCloskey J, Bulechek G. *Nursing Interventions Classification (NIC).* 2nd ed. St. Louis: Mosby Year Book; 1996.

National Council of State Boards of Nursing. Position Paper on the Licensure of Advanced Practice Nursing. Unpublished. 1992:1–8.

National League for Nursing. *Nursing Data Source.* New York: NLN; 1995.

Page N, Arena A. Rethinking the merger of the CNS and the NP roles. *Image.* 1994; 26(4): 315–318.

Rothberg J. The growth of political action in nursing. *Nurs Outlook.* 1985; 33:133–135.

Snyder M. *Independent Nursing Intervention.* Albany, NY: Delmar; 1992.

Spradley B, Dorsey B. Health of the home care population. In: Spradley B, ed. *Community Health Nursing Concepts and Practice.* 3rd ed. Glenview IL: Scott, Foresman/Little, Brown Higher Education; 1990:625–646.

Sweet J. Cost-effectiveness of nurse practitioners. *Nurs Econ.* 1986; 4:190–12.

U.S. Department of Health and Human Services. *The registered nurse population: Findings from the national sample of registered nurses,* March 1992. Washington, D.C., U.S. Government Printing Office; 1992.

Yura H, Walsh M. *The Nursing Process: Assessing, Planning, Implementing, Evaluating.* 5th ed. Norwalk, CT: Appleton & Lange; 1988.

BIBLIOGRAPHY

Adams C. Role expectations and role conflict of the army head nurse. *Nurs Manage.* 1988; 19(1):47–50.

American Nurses Association. *Nursing: A Social Policy Statement.* Kansas City, MO: ANA; 1980.

Aroian J, Rauckhorse L. Summer camp: An overlooked site for faculty clinical practice. *Nurse Educ.* 1985; 10(1):32–35.

Batra C. Socializing nurses for nursing entrepreneurship roles. *Nurs Health Care.* 1990; 11(1):35–37.

Felton G, Parsons MA, Satterfield P. Correctional facilities: A viable community health practice site for students. *J Community Health Nurs.* 1987; 4(2):111–115.

Ford L. A nurse for all settings, the nurse practitioner. *Nurs Outlook.* 1973; 23:381–384.

Loveridge C, Cummings S, O'Malley J. Developing case management in a primary nursing system. *J Nurs Admin.* 1988; 18(10):36–39.

McIntosh L. Hospital based case management. *Nurs Econ.* 1987; 5:232–236.

Pepe C. Surviving summer camp. *Can Nurse.* 1990; 86(4):18–21.

Terly B. Marketing private duty services. *Nurs Manage.* 1989; 20(3):57–59.

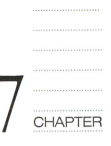

7
CHAPTER

Nursing Evaluation and Research

▸ **Objectives**

After studying the chapter the student will be able to:

1. Differentiate two methods of evaluation.
2. State examples of evaluation in terms of nursing practice and nursing education.
3. Define the components of research.
4. Identify trends in nursing research.
5. Explain how the research components remain vital to the discipline of nursing.
6. Discuss differences between quantitative and qualitative research methodologies.
7. Compare research methodology to the nursing process.

▸ **Questions to think about before reading the chapter**

- With what nursing research studies are you familiar?
- What are some areas of nursing research?
- Why is evaluation process an important part of nursing?
- Why is research in nursing needed?

▸ **Terms to know**

Accreditation	Evaluation
Analysis	Experimental research
Case-method research	Ex-post-facto research
Design	Field study research
Ethnographical research	Goal setting
Ethnoscience	Grounded theory studies

Historical research	Qualative research
Hypothesis	Quality assurance
Identification of area of interest	Quantitative research
Literature review	Reliability
National Institute for Nursing Research (NINR)	Research
Outcome evaluation	Scientific method
Phenomenological research	Structure evaluation
Postmodernism	Survey research
Process evaluation	Validity
Product evaluation	

▶ *Introduction*

Development of the discipline of nursing is based on theory, practice, and research. This chapter focuses on evaluation and nursing research. Evaluation and research are processes that may contribute to the life of an open system, since they are used to process input and information from the environment, produce findings, validate existing knowledge, or generate new information for continued life of the system. Evaluation and research are interrelated and form a circular process in which research provides criteria for evaluation and evaluation in turn raises questions for further research. They are processes by which data are organized, analyzed, and validated.

One purpose of this chapter is to provide an overview of evaluation and how it applies to nursing. Evaluation, as a component of the decision-making process, is discussed as it relates to client care and as an integral part of the nursing process, and also as it applies to nursing education and administration. Evaluation is part of a goal-directed process and is aimed at validation for maintenance of existing situations or for the promotion of change.

Other purposes of the chapter are to provide an overview of the research process and to discuss briefly the historical development of nursing research. Research contributes to nursing's body of knowledge through generation or validation of research questions or hypotheses. These, when validated, contribute to the knowledge base and science of nursing. The increase in knowledge that is generated by research may add to or validate existing nursing theory or generate new theory for the discipline. These theories provide direction for practice for the members of the discipline.

By using intellectual operations and contributing to nursing's body of knowledge, evaluation and research augment nursing's position as a profession and contribute to nursing's practice. This chapter is intended to provide a gen-

eral overview of these concepts and their relevance to the discipline of nursing. It is not its intent to discuss evaluation in depth or to teach research methodology.

EVALUATION

Evaluation, as a component of the decision-making process, is integral to the practice of nursing. Evaluation can be defined as the process of gathering information regarding attainment of specific organizational or individual goals and objectives. It is based on observable or measurable data. In making an evaluation, one must consider the values inherent in a situation, the criteria set for goal attainment, the process for achieving the goals, and the available resources. Personal and group values must be considered since they affect one's perception of a situation and thus affect the evaluative process. For example, a weight chart may indicate that a person's desired weight should be 160 pounds. The person losing weight may not value what has been given as expected weight. Thus, the difference in values may affect the criteria for evaluation of the outcome of the diet in terms of the client's weight change.

There are a variety of evaluative approaches; however, two types of evaluation are used in nursing, in the health care delivery system, and in nursing education. These are:

- Outcome, process, and structure evaluation
- Formative and summative evaluation

Evaluation must be planned rather than tacked on as an afterthought. Although there are many models for evaluation, usually three components are included: inputs, processes, and products (Friesner, 1978). The context of the situation or program being evaluated must also be considered.

One approach to evaluation used commonly in health and nursing is the outcome, process, and structure model. Meeting the criteria set for goal attainment (outcome or product), the methods for achieving the goals (process), and the available resources (structure) may be evaluated within this framework.

Another model for evaluation is the formative-summative model. Formative evaluation is the collection of information for assessment during the planning and implementing phases of an activity. Summative evaluation is assessment at the completion of an activity. All aspects of evaluation are considered at each of these times.

Evaluation in Nursing Care Situations

Outcome or **product evaluation.** Outcome or product evaluation, as it relates to nursing care, reflects on the actual behaviors or responses of the person after a plan of care has been completed. This plan of care is determined using the nursing process, as described in Chapter 3. Client goals and criteria are established to direct nursing care. The client-centered goals established for meeting client needs determine the outcome criteria. For example, it may be determined by the nurse and a new father and mother that the parents have a knowledge deficit related to infant care. One goal of the new parents might be to demonstrate giving a bath to their infant. The nurse, after having taught the bathing procedure, would observe the parents to determine if the goal of infant bathing had been met (outcome). A measurable goal for this situation would be: Parents will perform an infant bath, according to the procedure demonstrated by the nurses, before the infant is discharged from the hospital. Product evaluation is based on client statements and observable or measurable information about the client regarding the goal. Data collected from the client become the basis for assessing a new or additional nursing diagnosis or validating whether the stated diagnosis has been addressed.

Effectiveness of nursing care is determined by strict attainment goals and is measured by the evaluative process. Through the evaluative process, persons are held accountable for their actions by meeting the preset criteria or stating the rationale for not attaining the goal. Outcome or product evaluation as it relates to other areas of nursing is discussed later in this chapter.

Process Evaluation

In **process evaluation,** nursing actions are examined. This type of evaluation refers directly to nursing care. Process evaluation is important when client goals have been met but essential when client goals have not been achieved or have been only partially achieved. It is important when goals have been met to assess whether the particular interventions were best to meet the stated goal. However, it is essential when goals have not been completely achieved to determine the reason. Some possible reasons for not meeting the goal are inadequate intervention to meet the goal, inaccurate carrying out of nursing actions, or an inaccurate nursing diagnosis. In the previous example, process evaluation involves reflection on the actual intervention of teaching the bath procedure. If the parents could not adequately return the bath demonstration, the nurse would assess whether each step in the demonstration was included in the teaching; whether a bath demonstration was appropriate to meet the deficit in knowledge of infant care; whether the nursing diagnosis, knowledge deficit, was correct; or if another diagnosis, such as anxiety related to care of a newborn, would have been more appropriate. Such evaluation helps to determine whether the specific interventions need to be altered or a different diagnosis is necessary.

Another example of process evaluation is examination of specific nursing actions in a community health setting. A community health nurse may observe that a normally developing child has lost interest in eating. The nurse may identify a goal that includes an intake of specific amounts of vegetables or fruits, meat, and dairy equivalents each day. There are several approaches that may be selected to achieve the goal One approach may be to offer several small feedings throughout the day without verbal emphasis on the child's lack of eating. Another approach may be to develop a teaching plan for the parent concerning nutritional needs of the child and a plan for achieving these needs in terms of change in family eating practices and routines, with a referral to a dietitian. Both approaches may achieve the goal of having the child eat. However, in the first example, the approach is based on theory related to growth and development, while the approach in the second example is based on the teaching–learning theory. Evaluation of the approaches used in achieving the goal is process evaluation. Another aspect of process evaluation is whether the nurse was able to carry out the established plan of care.

Structure Evaluation

Structure evaluation is the way in which a system is constructed. Evaluation as applied to structure refers to obtaining feedback on resources in the environment, such as:

- Numbers and types of nursing personnel
- Financial resources
- Unit supplies
- Organizational structures
- Policies
- Procedures

Structure evaluation in a client care situation might relate to the number of staff available and their levels of educational preparation. In the initial example of the parents with a knowledge deficit related to infant care, availability of bath supplies and adequate numbers of nursing staff to carry out the plan are components to be considered in structural evaluation. In the second example, the community nurse evaluates for the type and availability of educational supplies and the caseload of the community health nurse. Effects of the environment on the system are also a part of the evaluation of structure.

This aspect of evaluation is based on expectations of others in the system related to what is needed to provide "quality" client care.

Evaluation and Quality Assurance

Evaluation may be applied to direct client care as well as to other areas that indirectly affect client care. The evaluative process is used by nurse administrators in various health care settings as part of quality assurance programs. **Quality assurance** is an organizational structure for evaluation of client care services. Nurse participation in quality assurance consists of several elements:

- Establishing a written plan of care based on health assessment
- Observing a situation, client, or nurse for the purposes of obtaining feedback
- Obtaining feedback from the client
- Documenting nursing actions and client responses (which commonly center around client problems and interventions to solve these problems)
- Measuring nursing care against preset standards of practice (nursing audit). The nursing audit generates a statement of overall quality nursing care

As indicated, nursing audit is one method of quality assurance. A nursing audit often includes a review of client records, peer review, and direct observation of client care. In the review of client care records, a nurse validates that predetermined goals of care have been met as documented in the client record. Peer review is evaluation of nurses by other nurses. It provides a system of accountability necessary to nursing in meeting professional criteria.

Evaluation and Nursing Education

Nursing education has been mentioned as an area in which evaluation is commonly used. The evaluative process is comprehensive and is used to determine the adequacy of the educational programs in preparing graduates for nursing practice. The process involves both the learner and the educator. The outcome or product, process, and structure model is often used for program evaluation. Outcome evaluation reflects whether the graduate has met program objectives on completion of the program of nursing studies. Often data are collected through questionnaires to the graduate and the agency employing the graduate. Process evaluation involves curriculum design and implementation. Students are an integral part of process evaluation. For example, students evaluate their own progress in meeting course objectives. They also evaluate faculty performance and course offerings. Several examples of what might be included in process evaluation are: the currency of the philosophy upon which the curriculum is designed, the method of delivery of instruction; and the sequence of courses in the program. Structure evaluation of a nursing program includes environmental factors (facilities, educational media, financial resources) and availability of quality administrators, faculty, and other support staff.

Use of a formative-summative evaluation model may be preferred in particular instances. For instance, it may be desirable to apply formative evaluation techniques with a newly developing curriculum or aspect of curriculum as it is being conceived and implemented. Summative evaluation techniques are applied once the curriculum or part of a curriculum has been implemented to determine progress toward stated goals.

Another type of evaluation commonly discussed in nursing education is norm- and criterion-referenced evaluation. In norm-referenced evaluation, a student's performance is compared against an established or standardized norm group. In criterion-referenced evaluation, minimum levels of expectation are established. A student's achievement is measured according to these preset standards.

Evaluation and Accreditation

A final means of using the evaluation process is through accreditation boards. **Accreditation** involves a voluntary process, in that institutions demonstrate their meeting of preset criteria. For example, one program objective for a baccalaureate nursing program might be that "the graduate will have the basis for graduate study in nursing"; another might be that "the graduate will be prepared as a beginning practitioner of professional nursing"; and a third might be that "the graduate will be prepared to contribute as an active member of society." An accrediting agency would ask for documentation of the graduate's ability to enter into and complete graduate study.

Many agencies accredit health care facilities and health educational programs. The National League for Nursing (NLN) is the official accrediting body for nursing education and community health nursing programs. The purpose of the accreditation process is to provide the public with a means to select quality nursing programs, to ensure qualified faculty and sound program design, to educate persons to be well prepared in nursing, and to provide continuous upgrading of nursing programs. Another example of an accrediting agency is the Joint Commission on Accreditation of Health Care Organizations (JCAHO), which accredits hospitals and nursing services for the purpose of documenting "quality" care. In addition, health care facilities must meet accreditation certification and reimbursement criteria for such programs as Medicare and Medicaid.

RESEARCH

The development of nursing research can be thought of as following the components of structure, process, and outcome. Early research focused on structures within nursing, such as types of nursing programs, availability of nurses, and areas of nursing practice. The trend in research developed toward process, in which nurses studied other nurses, students, and learning processes. In the mid to late 1970s, nursing research was oriented toward quasi experimental approaches and focused on patient care in terms of process and outcome. The emphasis was on the results of nursing interventions and not only the interventions themselves. This has been frequently referred to as "clinical research." Historical research was also being conducted at this time. Currently, nursing research has expanded from historical and quasi experimental designs to include other methods of qualitative and quantitative design. Areas of study of nursing research have also expanded to include theory testing and nurse-client situations.

Research is a systematic process based on certain constraints and expectations. It tests hypotheses and theories, or generates new ideas and hypotheses. Research involves studies of presumed relationships by means of hypothetical question and studies of phenomena of interest to the investigator. Research must be expressed in terms of meaning to the reader for it to be of use as a means for building and advancing knowledge. Currently there are many types of research. These include quantitative and qualitative research. **Quantitative research** refers to an objective, deductive methodology that enables the investigator to count or number the phenomena of interest in order to apply statistical tests to the data. **Qualitative research** is a descriptive, inductive investigation of an area of concern without the use of numbering or counting. Some examples of quantitative research are **historical** (interpretations of past events); **survey** (use of questionnaires, polls, etc.); **case-method** (analysis of causation and interrelationships); **experimental** (controlled experiment in which at least one causative factor is manipulated and randomization is used); and **ex-post-facto research** (data are collected after the event has occurred and therefore cannot be manipulated) (Brill & Kilts, 1980; Kerlinger, 1986). Examples of qualitative research methods are historical; **field study** (observation of people in their everyday environment); **grounded theory studies** (data grounded in fact and theory generated from the theory), **ethnographical** (observation documenting and analyzing life patterns of a culture to gain insight into the people within their own environment), and **phenomenological** (analysis of the descriptions of experiences to determine the essence of the experience). These research methods involve the use of key informants, secondary informants, and participant-observer methods of data collection.

DeGroot (1988) identified major factors that influence scientific research in nursing. These are intrapersonal and extrapersonal factors. Intrapersonal factors include:

- Individual's world view (i.e., nature of human beings, nature of knowledge and truth, and nature of nursing science)
- Cognitive style (i.e., person's usual mode of thinking, perceiving, and solving problems)
- Experience encompassing life experience, professional nursing experience, research experience, and theoretical experiences
- Methodological knowledge and skill

Extrapersonal factors include influential others and sociohistorical context. DeGroot states that all of these factors or variables relate, interact, and influence each other. Changes in one variable impact on many other variables or factors in nursing research.

Format

As previously stated, research is a systematic approach to the development of knowledge and testing or validation of theory. It can involve hypothesis-testing or hypothesis-producing methods. The research process is the approach used to investigate the phenomena or area of inquiry. The process used (i.e., qualitative or quantitative) is based on individual definitions of research, the direction of research, and the formulation of the area of interest. The process chosen helps to define the methodology that the researcher will follow. The methodology used also helps to define the process. For example, if the research process uses the **scientific method** (a systematic, controlled, observable investigation based on theory) approach to research (quantitative), steps that may be taken are:

- Identification of the problem
- Review of the literature
- Development of the theoretical framework
- Identification of the variables
- Statement of the hypotheses
- Determination of the methodology
- Collection and analysis of data
- Report of the findings

If the **ethnoscience** process (a systematic way of studying from within a culture that particular culture's perceptions of its own universe) is used (qualitative), the steps may be identified as (Leininger, 1985):

- Identification of the key informants
- Interview
- Community involvement
- Group data coding
- Verification and validation of impressions with informants
- Report of the findings

There are many processes that are encompassed by research.

Regardless of the approach used, the research process is a specialized problem-solving one. It is specialized in that the question, problem or concern, or area of interest is studied in a defined and systematic way that has been agreed upon by others. The process must meet specified criteria and standards of reliability and validity established by the chosen research methodology. **Validity** and **reliability** are defined in different ways, depending on the research method used. Leininger (1985) states that the aim of criteria of validity and reliability in quantitative research is on ensuring that the instruments and measurements used in research measure what is intended and do it consistently and accurately. The aim of qualitative validity and reliability, according to Leininger, is to confirm the truth or understanding of the phenomenon under investigation and the consistency of the study to reveal meaningful and accurate truths about a phenomenon. Thus, the focus is on the phenomenon being studied and not on the instruments or measurements of the phenomenon as in quantitative research. Problem solving can be viewed as the umbrella concept, and research process is a very specialized, systematic part of that process.

Newman (1982) draws parallels between the stages of the research design, themes of inquiry in nursing research, and levels of theory for a profession. She states that, although the fit of these three levels may not be perfect, it provides a sense of the ongoing process of research and theory development and "connects the levels of theory with the appropriate research design and content as well as the ultimate purpose of nursing theory (i.e., application in practice)" (p. 87). For further discussion on theory development, see Chapter 1.

There are basic steps to be followed to complete the research process. The basic steps are:

- Identification of the area of interest
- Goal setting or hypothesis stating
- Review of current knowledge in the area
- Design of the study
- Analysis or coding of the findings
- Discussion of the findings

These steps are not necessarily conducted in the order presented here. The methodology selected is dependent on many factors, such as:

- The researcher's philosophy
- The area of concern or interest
- The purpose of the research
- The statement or research question
- Researcher experience
- Costs
- Ethical considerations
- The proposed use of the findings

Human subjects review boards are used to ensure that ethical concerns are addressed by the researcher and the design used for the study. Ethical considerations in nursing are considered further in Chapter 8.

Identification of Area of Interest

Identification of area of interest generally occurs as a result of an "educated hunch," from direct observation of situations, gaps in knowledge, or controversy. It may also result from unanswered questions from other research findings or from interest in a particular phenomenon that has not yet been adequately investigated. For example, the nurse researcher may wonder what the concept of health means to people in other cultures or in an American subculture. Or perhaps the nurse notices that in a particular setting, when soft music is playing, clients request less pain medication. From these observations or curious probing into phenomena of interest, the researcher develops a preliminary area of interest for investigation.

Goal Setting or Hypothesis Formation

All research is conducted for a specific purpose. **Goals** are set or **hypotheses** are identified to determine specific factors or relationships to be investigated and to explicate the purpose of the research. In research, either the research question or the statement of the hypothesis determines the type of statistical analysis to be used to evaluate the data. The research question or hypothesis includes main factors to be studied or variables to be included. For example, the goal of a qualitative research project may be to determine the concept of care in a Greek population in Detroit, Michigan. In a quantitative research project, the researcher may be interested in the relationship of the variables of stress and age on women's health.

Review of Current Knowledge in the Area

The researcher must be knowledgeable about current developments in the area of interest. Information is gathered in a **literature review.** The review of literature in quantitative designs is used to determine previous studies in the area, to determine significant findings obtained by previous investigations, and to validate the problem statement. This prevents unnecessary duplication of previous research findings and establishes the need for further research.

Qualitative research sometimes involves a literature search. In some types of qualitative research, such as grounded research, this search is conducted after the study has been completed; other qualitative research methods require literature reviews prior to data collection. The qualitative researcher who is conducting research in another culture must be thoroughly familiar with the language, cultural beliefs, and practices of that culture. This is required to study the phenomena adequately from the point of view of the people within that culture and not from the investigator's point of view.

Design of Study

The **design** of the research project is dependent on the type of research being conducted, the problem being studied, or the statement of hypotheses. It specifies the population to be used and the methods for collecting data. The sample must be specific to the problem and representative of the population. For example, in quantitative research, the sample of college freshmen in 60 universities across the country may be representative of all college freshmen in the United States if the sample was randomly selected and the number (60) was sufficient for concluding that the results of the study could not have happened by chance alone. In qualitative research, eight or ten key informants and 30 or 40 secondary informants may be representative of the population of Australian aborigines, since the use of the findings does not involve statistical manipulation, there is intense interviewer involvement, and revalidation of the findings is done with every informant. The methods used for collecting the data in all research must not cause harm to the subjects and data must be collected with the consent of the participants. Every researcher must follow specific guidelines to ensure that human subjects' rights are not violated. This includes the ensurance of informed consent, freedom from harm, and privacy, anonymity, and confidentiality. There are many methods to collect data (e.g., historical documents, letters, questionnaires, surveys, physiological equipment, participant-observer interviews).

Analysis or Coding of Data

In quantitative research, **analysis** may follow specific statistical rules to determine to what extent the hypotheses were supported. In qualitative research, the data are coded to determine patterns and specific cultural usages. In this step of the research process, the researcher determines the significance of the data and applies the analysis to the hypothesis or goals identified at the start of the project. Significance in quantitative methodology implies specific statistical testing to determine what percent of the total is necessary to accept or fail to accept the hypothesis. Significance in qualitative research is the significance that the concept or area of interest has to the population being studied and any implications for further research.

Discussion of the Findings

The findings of the research project must indicate what was found as a result of the investigation. In quantitative research, the findings must indicate the extent to which the hypothesis was supported. The discussion of the findings indicates the biases of the study and the major conclusions. The findings suggest areas for future investigation and research and have implications for nursing practice, education, and administration.

All research must be read critically to assess the validity of the findings and the importance of the results. All the steps of the project need to be analyzed to ensure that the study has been adequately conducted and that the specific methodology has been used.

Historical Focus of Nursing Research

Nursing uses the methodology described to study issues relevant to the discipline. Nursing research must be based on phenomena of interest to the discipline. It may be oriented to practice, theory, or the generation of knowledge.

Munhall and Oiler (1986) describe three contextual events that have led to the expansion of nursing research. One event is that since around the middle of the century there has been a change in the theoretical approaches to viewing and understanding phenomena in many fields. For instance, systems theory, described in Chapter 2, has been widely used in recent years as a means of viewing phenomena from a broad perspective. The rapid rise in technological advances and the scientific knowledge explosion precipitated the need to manage and manipulate large data bases. Nursing responded to societal change, as well as to its own internal needs for professional development. The need for recognition as a profession with a distinct body of nursing knowledge led to theory development using nursing models. This theoretical development of nursing and the changes in world views or paradigms have been discussed in more detail in Chapter 1.

A second event in the expansion of nursing research is the education of doctorally prepared nurses in areas outside nursing, since doctoral education in nursing has only recently begun to develop. (See Chapter 3.) Since the mid-20th century, there has been heavy emphasis on quantitative research using predominantly the scientific method. More recently, qualitative research is being employed in response to the limitations of the scientific approach in addressing some of nursing's phenomena. The third event in expansion of nursing research is that nurses who were educated in fields outside nursing have conducted research studies based on frameworks in the language of their doctoral field (e.g., sociology, anthropology, education).

It is important to emphasize that this change in approach to nursing, along with the recent growth in number of nurses with doctor's degrees, has resulted in an increased expansion of nursing research, both quantitative and qualitative. There is an increasing number of nurses knowledgeable about the research process and the use of research in the development of nursing.

Nursing research also provides an element of accountability for decisions made in practice. The consumer movement has forced accountability of actions for health providers. The rising cost of health care and the active participation of consumers in health care are forcing nurses to ask if nursing actions are effective and if they make a difference. Research helps to determine the effectiveness of the interventions used in the nursing process and the results of the interventions generate questions for future nursing research. Research is also conducted for expansion of knowledge in nursing in areas other than practice. Research is performed around concepts related to nursing theories and areas of nursing concern. This advances the profession and assists in the establishment of the uniqueness of nursing as a discipline.

When we view nursing historically, certain issues become apparent. Florence Nightingale is considered an early researcher, since many of her reforms, such as the changes in environmental and sanitation conditions in hospitals, were based on investigation. Although Florence Nightingale engaged in beginning research activity, nursing research did not develop in America. Nursing schools in America at the turn of the century did not support critical thinking or problem-solving skills (Donahue, 1985). This may have been due to the apprenticeship nature of nursing education. "Training schools" at that time did not encourage research or evaluation of nursing care. Information was passed on by word of mouth and was not based on scientific knowledge. Research grew slowly because women were not well educated and their role at that time inhibited the asking of questions. As women's status and educational opportunities improved, so did nursing. The development of schools of nursing within universities resulted in more opportunity for and awareness of the need for research.

Even though the opportunities for nursing research were slow to develop, many nursing leaders recognized the need for research in nursing. In 1912, one leader, M. Adelaide Nutting, studied nursing educational conditions after the turn of the century. Her findings—that the conditions under which nurses functioned were appalling—were published in "The Educational Status of Nursing" (Nutting, 1912).

Another nursing leader in the 1920s was Isabel M. Stewart. She investigated the use of time and motion studies for nursing and began to differentiate between nursing and nonnursing tasks. She also published the *Nursing Education Bulletin,* an early research journal in nursing (Donahue, 1985).

Research studies conducted in the 1920s were concerned with nursing education, problems with staffing on the units, and comparisons of students from different programs. Subsequent research in the 1930s and 1940s was based on the industrial management model, with the focus on nurses in studies similar to the popular industrial time and motion studies. In addition, hospital staffing patterns and nursing education were also subjects for research.

The Second World War created an increased need for nurses. Nursing research became centered around the number of nurses in practice and the areas of need created by the nursing shortage. The Brown Report of 1948 gave impetus to research studies aimed at functions, attitudes and roles of nurses; hospital settings; and patient interactions (Abdellah & Levine, 1965).

The 1950s brought an increase in the number of nurses with advanced educational preparation. Baccalaureate and master's degree programs in nursing were developing, and many research methodology courses were incorporated in the curriculums. The increase in educational preparation of nurses placed greater emphasis on nursing research. The once-small number of educated researchers is increasing as a result of the increased number of nurses earning doctoral degrees.

Research of the 1950s focused on nurses in practice and how society and other health professionals viewed nursing. The journal *Nursing Research* was first published in 1952 in response to the increased awareness of the need. In 1955, the American Nurses' Foundation was established. Its main purpose was to further nursing research and encourage its continuance. The first United States Public Health Service awards for nursing research also were given in 1956. Prior to the establishment of doctoral programs in nursing, a federal program to educate nurses in research methodology was established. These "nurse scientists" received doctoral preparation in nurse-related fields such as anthropology, philosophy, sociology, and physiology. Graduates of these programs were able to apply research methodology to areas of nursing. Even though nurse scientists applied research to nursing, their major emphasis was on the theoretical concepts based on nonnursing frameworks. Since then, there has been an increase in the number of nurses who have earned degrees within doctoral nursing programs. The increase in nursing theory development and nurse doctorates has expanded nursing theory research based in nursing frameworks.

As discussed previously, the impetus for nursing theory development occurred during the 1960s. Research changed its central focus, and nurses began to study outcomes of nursing care rather than nurses themselves. Lysaught's *Abstract for Action* (1970) increased nursing attention to the importance of studying the effects of nursing interventions and quality of care. The recommendations from this study reinforced the need for evaluation and quality nursing research.

In the American Nurses Association (ANA) study of 1974, the ANA stated that the primary concern of nursing research should be developing nursing practice, testing nursing theories, documenting patient outcomes, and evaluating effectiveness of nursing interventions. The shift in nursing research has been from studying the education of nurses, curriculum designs, and nursing actions to study of patient outcomes of nursing interventions. With an increase in nursing research, the knowledge basis of nursing continues to develop.

In 1985, Congress established a National Institute of Health having a National Center for Nursing Research (NCNR). In 1993 the NCNR was redesignated the **National Institute of Nursing Research (NINR).** The mission of the NINR is "to promote science that strengthens nursing practice and improves health care. NINR supports interdisciplinary research and research training in universities, hospitals, and research centers across the country and conducts intramural investigations at NIH" (NINR WWW homepage, 1996).

Qualitative research in nursing also began gaining acceptance in the 1980s. Before this time, nurses were concerned with developing nursing knowledge by means of scientific research methodology. This was considered necessary in the struggle for nursing to attain the status of a scientific discipline. Current nursing authors are questioning the sole use of the scientific method to develop all of nursing's knowledge, since many questions in nursing can no longer be answered by solely using a quantitative approach. One point of view is that nursing should move to a larger world view and a new way of viewing phenomena (Munhall & Oiler, 1986).

Many nurses believe that qualitative and quantitative research are of equal value in the development of nursing knowledge. Many authors (Chinn, 1985; Fawcett, 1984; Gorenberg, 1983; Polit & Hungler, 1983; Tinkle & Beaton, 1983; Tripp-Reimer, 1985; Watson, 1985) advocate the use of these two methodologies together to advance nursing knowledge. It is suggested that these methods complement each other in terms of types of knowledge derived from each approach. Quantitative methodology is recommended for use in verifying knowledge, testing hypotheses, and generalizing to large populations. Qualitative research is recommended for generating hypotheses, understanding relationships, and illustrating the meaning of descriptions and relationships.

Greene (1979) and others suggest that quantitative research be used for the scientific aspects of nursing while qualitative research addresses the art of nursing. This forced dichotomy has also created problems for researchers. The quantitative-method paradigm can be incorporated into the qualitative paradigm by various means.

Nursing's knowledge advancement depends on the ability of nurses to find the right questions for research and the best means of answering these questions. Qualitative research can provide the context of meaning in which quantitative findings can be understood (Filstead, 1983). Goodwin & Goodwin (1983) advocate appropriate use of both methodologies in order to achieve a comprehensiveness that neither alone can achieve and to cross-validate findings.

Philipps (1990) states that "research should focus on ... the study of people's experiencing of their health, their sense of interconnectedness with others and specifically, how health emerges from a mutual process." In 1995 he stated that global nursing is an expanding area for nursing research with the potential to open new attitudes and values for nursing. He emphasized that nursing knowledge is not permanent or written in stone but will be transformed by global nursing research to become a nursing science of wholeness that is much more diverse than what we now know.

Both qualitative and quantitative paradigms and resultant processes can address similar purposes, aims, and goals; show some rigor in methodology used; advance human knowledge as well as nursing knowledge; address concepts of person, environment, and health; and be used together or separately. To ignore one means of developing knowledge is to ignore the aim of knowledge discovery. These paradigms have overlapping gray areas where the methodologies may intertwine. For example, both qualitative and quantitative paradigms use descriptive fieldwork and interviewing. They must be viewed independently as well as interdependently in order to advance nursing knowledge.

Rogers (1994) does not totally agree with this view. She states that we make a big mistake by trying to categorize everything. This is a western world view of life. She states that research needs to look at the phenomenon under study and determine the best ways to understand it rather than mix together whatever methodologies we have that will answer the question with the least amount of effort and cost. Rogers does not believe that applied research provides new knowledge, it only tests knowledge that is already available. This is not productive to building nursing knowledge for human betterment, according to Rogers.

Watson (1995) describes the **postmodernism** view in terms of nursing. This view is an extension of the works of Rogers in the sense that postmodernism represents the end of the western mind-set, with the dominance of one way of viewing reality, or one world view. Watson describes postmodernistic thinking as the beginning and the end of modernity.

She points out that postmoderism is the contrast to positivist reasoning, where knowledge equals science which equals reality. The postmodernist view allows for many realities existing at one time. Many authors (Fawcett 1984; Newman, 1986, 1991; Parse 1989; Rogers 1994) have written extensively on the need to examine differing philosophical understandings beyond the logical positivist world view in which everything can be explained by cause and effect in a linear world. This has great impact on the way research is viewed, conducted, and explained.

Research and Practice

Nursing research is essential for the development and evaluation of nursing practice. Abu-Saad (1993) stresses that nursing research generates information for practice that helps nurses understand human health-related experiences. She states that nursing research should not develop in a vacuum.

Crow (1982) suggests four approaches to nursing research in order to enhance its contribution to practice. These approaches are research to:

1. Provide insights into practice.
2. Deepen one's understanding of concepts central to care.
3. Develop new or improved methods of caring.
4. Test the effectiveness of the care given.

Research that provides insights into practice focuses on studies specific to patient practices and means of interviewing in these practices. Research to deepen understanding of concepts of care nurses plan to deliver involves such concepts as pain, anxiety, sleep, infections, and role. Research to develop new or improved methods of care is self-evident. The fourth approach looks at care practices in order to determine the effectiveness of nursing care. This type of research parallels the focus in outcome evaluation. Crow states the significance of nursing research will be determined by the impact it makes on the health care needs of the community.

Nursing research provides the basis for change in nursing interventions and improvement of health care for consumers through the study of culture, psychology, physiology, and social concepts, with an emphasis on health (Brill & Kilts, 1980; Ellis, 1977; Leininger, 1976). The increased awareness of the need for nursing research has resulted in research courses being offered in undergraduate nursing programs and research studies conducted in graduate level nursing programs. Nurses are specializing in nursing research and helping to promote research in various institutions. All nurses can play a role in research, even though all nurses do not conduct research. Research is directly related to identified problems for which nurses are responsible and that affect nursing care of clients and nurses themselves.

Research provides a means to evaluate the nursing care given to clients, and provides new methods and ideas for the improvement of nursing care. It is vital to the improvement of client health conditions and to assure that nursing will continue to meet the criteria of a profession. Nurses, as researchers, contribute to the expansion of health care and promotion of health to society through collaboration with researchers in other health disciplines and sharing of research findings.

Research is a problem-solving process of inquiry. Basic research is conducted to generate knowledge; applied research seeks practical means for utilizing that knowledge. The nursing process is a scientific process that closely follows the guidelines of research methodology and applied research. It involves the identification of a health state or potential or actual problem, review of literature through interpretation of data collected by assessment, and methodology or nursing intervention to meet the identified problem or need. It also includes evaluation of the methodology to determine if the need was met. While the nursing process does not strictly follow the steps of research methodology, it does follow an established systematic process.

The evaluation process is different from the research process. Evaluation involves a systematic means of determine the effect of a technique, program, or change elicited by an intervention or a procedure. Evaluation can occur as a result of knowledge gained by the research process. It can stimulate a problem or area of concern that needs to be looked at by the researcher, and can have a circular interaction with the research process. Evaluation does not test theory or stimulate new knowledge; rather, it identifies areas of concern or validates changes or current situations. Evaluation research is an applied form of research, according to Polit & Hungler (1995). Its goal is to evaluate the success of a program, practice, or policy. The research process is the means of stimulating new knowledge and validating theories.

SUMMARY

Evaluation is essential to determine effectiveness, accountability, and professionalism in the discipline of nursing. It involves the components of values, criteria, and decision-making process. Structure-process-outcome and formative and summative evaluation are two common methods of evaluation. These methods can be applied to nursing, nursing administration, and nursing education. Nursing research provides a basis for the development of theory and broadens the body of knowledge. It also contributes to the improvement of nursing practice. As nursing research continues to validate theory, the quality of care will improve as a result of the expanded basis for decision making. Research also assists with movement of nursing toward professionalization and establishment of the uniqueness of the discipline. Nursing process has been related to scientific research methodology. As nursing researchers collaborate with researchers from other health professions, health care delivery to consumers will improve.

▶ Questions for Discussion

1. Discuss the methods of evaluation.
2. Compare differences in formative and summative evaluation.
3. How does evaluation relate to research?
4. Why is nursing research important?
5. What trends have occurred in nursing research?
6. Compare research to the nursing process.
7. What are differences and similarities between qualitative and quantitative research?
8. How are nursing research, nursing theory, and nursing practice related?

REFERENCES

Abdellah F, Levine E. *Better Patient Care through Nursing Research.* New York: Macmillan; 1965.

Abu-Saad HH 1993; Nursing the science and the practice. *Int J Nurs Stud.* 30(3); 287–294.

American Nurses Association. Resolutions of priorities in nursing research. *Am Nurs.* 1974; 6:5.

Bril EL, Kilts DF. *Foundations for Nursing.* New York: Appleton-Century-Crofts; 1980.

Chinn P. Debunking the myths in nursing theory and research. *Image.* 1985; 17(2):45–49.

Crow R. How nursing and the community can benefit from nursing research. *Int J Nurs Stud.* 1982; 19(1):37–45.

DeGroot H. Scientific inquiry in nursing: A model for a new age. *Adv Nurs Sci.* 1988; 10(3):1–21.

Donahue MP. *Nursing, the Finest Art.* St. Louis: Mosby; 1985.

Ellis R. Fallibilities, fragments and frames: Contemplating on 25 years in medical/surgical nursing. *Nurs Res.* 1977; 26:177–182.

Fawcett J. Hallmarks of success in nursing research. *Adv Nurs Res.* 1984; 7(1):1–11.

Filstead W. Qualitative method: A needed perspective in evaluation research. In: Cook T, Reichardt C, eds. *Qualitative and Quantitative Methods in Evaluation Research.* Beverly Hills, CA: Sage Publications; 1983.

Friesner A. Five models for program evaluation: An overview. In: Yura H, Friesner A, King DC, eds. *Curriculum Process for Developing and Revising Baccalaureate Nursing Programs* (NLN publication # 15-1700). New York: National League for Nursing; 1978.

Goodwin L, Goodwin W. Qualitative vs. quantitative research or qualitative and quantitative research? *Nurs Res.* 1983; 32:347–349.

Gorenberg B. An emerging issue. *Nurs Res.* 1983; 32:347–349.

Greene J. Science, nursing, and nursing science: A conceptual analysis. *Adv Nurs Sci.* 1979; 2(1):57–64.

Kerlinger F. *Foundations of Behavioral Research.* 3rd ed. New York: Holt, Rinehart, & Winston; 1986.

Leininger M. Doctoral programs for nurses. Trends, questions and projected plans. *Nurs Res.* 1976; 25:201–210.

Leininger M. Ethnography and ethnonursing: Models and modes of qualitative data analysis. In: Leininger M, ed. *Qualitative Research Methods in Nursing.* Orlando, Fla.: Grune & Stratton; 1985.

Lysaught J. *An Abstract for Action.* New York: McGraw-Hill; 1970.

Munhall P, Oiler C. *Nursing Research: A Qualitative Approach.* Norwalk CT: Appleton-Century-Crofts; 1986.

Newman M. Health as expanding consciousness. St. Louis: Mosby; 1986.

Newman M. What differentiates clinical research. *Image.* 1982; 14(3): 86–88.

Newman M, Sime AM, Corcoran-Perry SA. The focus of the discipline of nursing. *Adv Nurs Sci.* 1991; 14(1):1–6.

Nutting MA. Educational status of nursing. *U.S. Bureau of Education Bulletin.* 1912; 7.

Parse, RR. Man-living-health: a theory of nursing. In: J. Riehl-Sisca (ed.). *Conceptual Models for Nursing Practice.* 3rd ed. Norwalk, CT: Appleton & Lange; 1989.

Phillips JR. The different views of health. *Nurs Sci Q.* 1990; 3(3):103–104.

Phillips JR. Martha Rogers' clarion call for global nursing research. *Nurs Sci Q.* 1995; 7(3):100–101.

Phillips JR. Nursing theory-based research for advanced nursing practice. *Nurs Sci Q.* 1995; 8(1):4–5.

Polit D, Hungler B. *Nursing Research: Principles and Methods.* 5th ed. Philadelphia: Lippincott; 1995.

Rogers M. The science of unitary human beings: Current perspectives. *Nurs Sci Q.* 1994; 7(1):33–35.

Tinkle M, Beaton J. Toward a new view of science: Implications for nursing research. *Adv Nurs Sci.* 1983; 5(2):27–36.

Tripp-Reimer T. Combining qualitative and quantitative methodologies. In: Leininger M, ed. *Qualitative Research Methods in Nursing.* Orlando, FL: Grune & Stratton; 1985.

Watson J. Postmodernism and knowledge development in nursing. *Nurs Sci Q.* 1995; 8(2):60–64.

Watson J. Reflections on different methodologies for the future of nursing. In: Leininger M, ed. *Qualitative Research Methods in Nursing.* Orland, FL: Grune & Stratton; 1985.

BIBLIOGRAPHY

American Nurses' Association. Resolutions of priorities in nursing research. *Am Nurse.* 1974; 6:5.

Armiger B. Ethics of nursing research: Profile, principles, perspective. *Nurs Res.* 1977; 26:330.

Benoliel JQ. The interaction between theory and research. *Nurs Outlook.* 1977; 25:108.

Brochet J. Historical photo-analysis: Research methodology. *Hist Methods.* 1982; 15(2):35–44.

Creighton H. Legal concerns of nursing research. *Nurs Res.* 1977; 26:337.

Chaska NL, ed. *The Nursing Profession: View Through the Mist.* New York: McGraw-Hill; 1978.

Cook T, Reichardt C, eds. *Qualitative and Quantitative Methods in Evaluation Research.* Beverly Hills, CA: Sage Publications; 1983.

Dickoff J, James P, Semradek J. 8-4 Research. Part 11. Designing nursing research-8 points of encounter. *Nurs Res.* 1975; 24:164–176.

Diers D. Application of research to nursing practice. *Image.* 1972; 5: 7–11.

Evers S. Nursing ethics: The central concept of nursing education. *Nurse Educ.* 1984; 9(3):14–18.

Froebe DJ, Bain R. *Quality Assurance Programs and Controls in Nursing.* St. Louis: Mosby; 1976.

Gortner SR, Nahm H. An overview of nursing research in the U.S. *Nurs Res.* 1977; 26:10–30.

Leininger M. *Qualitative Research Methods in Nursing.* Orland, FL: Grune & Stratton; 1985.

Mocca P. A critique of compromise: Beyond the methods debate. *Adv Nurs Sci.* 1988; 10(4): 1–9.

Myers S, Haase J. Guidelines for integration of quantitative and qualitative approaches. *Nurs Res.* 1989; 38(5):299–301.

Oiler C. The phenomenological approach in nursing research. *Nurs Res.* 1982; 31:178–181.

Phillips J. Qualitative research: A process of discovery. *Nurs Sci Q.* 1989; 5–6.

Sandelowski M. The problem of rigor in qualitative research. *Adv Nurs Sci.* 1986; 8(3):27–37.

Stem PN. Grounded theory methodology: Its uses and processes. *Image.* 1980; 12:20–23 .

Swanson J, Chenitz WC. Why qualitative research in nursing? *Nurs Outlook.* 1982; 30:241–244.

Swanson-Kauffinan K. A combined qualitative methodology for nursing research. *Adv Nurs Sci.* 1986; 8(3):58–69.

Wald F, Leonard R. Towards development of nursing practice theory. *Nurs Res.* 1964; 13:309.

8

CHAPTER

Ethical and Legal Considerations

After studying the chapter, the student will be able to:

1. Discuss three areas of ethical concern for nurses.
2. State two aspects of the decision-making process.
3. Identify two areas of legal concern to nurses.
4. Define the purpose of nurse practice acts.
5. Identify several ethical and legal dilemmas concerning nursing.

▶ **Questions to think about before reading the chapter**

- What ethical concerns of health care have you read or heard about?
- What is meant by a decision-making framework?
- Are you aware of any ethical problems related to nursing?
- What is the nurse practice act?
- What laws protect the consumers from individuals practicing nursing without the knowledge or skills required for such care?

▶ **Terms to know**

American Nurses Credentialing Center
  (ANCC)
Accreditation
Board of nursing
Certification
Civil law

Code of Ethics
Common law
Computer-adaptive testing (CAT)
Credentialing
Ethics
Informed consent

Laws

Liability

Licensure

Malpractice

Morals

National Council of State Boards of Nursing
(NCSBN)

NCLEX-RN (National Council Licensure
Examination-Registered Nurses)

Negligence

Nurse practice act

Registration

Statutory laws

▶ *Introduction*

The health care delivery system was presented in Chapter 5 as a complex, multi-disciplinary structure whose purpose is the maintenance of health and the provision of care to clients. Two areas essential for consideration in the provision of health and nursing care to the client are ethics and law. Knowledge of these areas is also important in the way it affects society and the health care professionals providing care. Nurses as health care providers are responsible for their actions and accountable for care given and judgments made. To maintain this accountability ethical and legal standards have been established by society, the consumer, the nursing profession, and other health care professionals.

Nurses and other health care professionals develop frameworks that serve as guides for ethical decision making. Such a framework in nursing includes identification of the nurse's own values and beliefs; the values and beliefs of clients; the goals of the profession and other professionals; and rights and responsibilities related to ethical decisions. A code of ethics is established by each profession as a guide for standards of practice.

Nursing responds to and has influence on societal health care needs. Laws govern nursing practice to protect society. Although legislators formulate laws, nurses must have input into this process. Nurses help create guidelines for acceptable and safe nursing practice. Legal guidelines are essential to safeguard the autonomy of the nursing profession.

This chapter highlights some ethical and legal concerns in nursing. To detail issues is not the intent here. Rather, it is to introduce the student to the implications of the issues. Ethical concerns relegate to client care situations, nursing practice, and the promotion of the professional discipline. Legal concerns are identified in relation to credentialing and nursing practice.

ETHICAL CONSIDERATIONS

The words *ethics* and *morals* are often used synonymously. However, some writers differentiate between them: morals indicate "the oughts and shoulds of society," and ethics indicate "the principles behind the shoulds" (Thompson & Thompson, 1981, p. 1). Together they provide standards and principles to guide conduct and decision making in the protection of human rights. Ethics are essential to all professions. They are based on the values and principles of a profession and are reflected in a profession's standards of practice.

A person's values are central to ethical decision making. Values are beliefs held concerning the worth, the truth, and the desirability of an idea, object, or behavior (Czmowski, 1974). These serve as guides for personal behavior. Values are derived from the individual's life experiences and the interpretation of these as well as the experiences of others. They form the basis for personal conduct, actions, and behavior (within which the individual performs and views the acts of others). Values are based on the background and culture of the individual. The values of the nurse, other health care professionals, and the client may differ.

An example of differing values related to health may be illustrated in the following situation:

> An elderly person who is living alone may value the right to make a decision regarding self-care in the home. The value may relate to belief in autonomy or the cultural belief that the elderly are to be cared for by the children. The children may value their own autonomy from the parent and the right to maintain a separate lifestyle. They may determine that the elderly parent is to be cared for in an extended-care facility. The health care professional may value either the elderly person's or the children's right to make the decision or may believe that the health care professional should be the one to make the decision. This belief may be based on the value that professional knowledge provides for a more accurate judgment. Ethics assist in determining which values will be considered in a given situation.

Professionals formulate values. The work of nursing has been the essence of ethics and ethical behavior, that of fostering good through nursing care and working to prevent harm through that same care. According to Donaldson and Crowley (1978), the value orientation of professional practice is to foster "self-care behavior that leads to individual health and well-being." Donaldson and Crowley also state that "As a result of this value orientation, knowledge of the basis of human choices and of methods for fostering individual independence are sought, rather than knowledge of interventions that control and directly manipulate the person per se into a societally determined state of health."

Persons develop frameworks by which to reason relative to moral decisions. These frameworks may include theories of ethics, intuition (a commonsense approach), a formal approach as with a professional code, and the conventional or sociological approach (Bandman & Bandman 1995). They identify some eleven theoretical approaches (Fig. 8–1). Each of these approaches emphasizes core values related to persons and society, rights and responsibilities, or aspects such as principles of goodness and happiness, justice and freedom that need to be considered when making ethical decisions. A conflict sometimes occurs when individuals or groups involved in

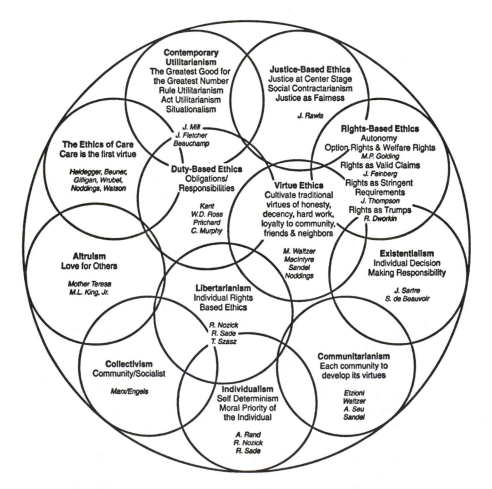

Figure 8–1. Contemporary ethical theories. Assume that they whirl around each other. *(From Bandman E, Bandman B. Nursing Ethics Through the Lifespan. 3rd ed. Appleton & Lange: Norwalk, CT; 1995.)*

the decision have theoretical approaches with differing core values. For instance, one person or group may value the right of the individual above all else while another may value most highly the needs of society.

Professionals develop codes of ethics and standards for practice to assist in decision making at the professional level. Codes and standards form a foundation for the evaluation of professional performance by the public and by other members of the professions. The American Nurses Association has formulated general and specialized standards of practice. The general standards of practice can be found in Chapter 1.

The American Nurses Association (ANA) also has formulated a **Code of Ethics,** which is reprinted here. A variety of themes may be identified in this code. Dignity of the client, including confidentiality and privacy, is one theme. Professional development, peer accountability, knowledge acquisition, and economic sanctions are other themes important to the professional nurse. The last two themes identified are protection of the public and collaboration with other health care professionals (Fenner, 1980).

CODE OF ETHICS FOR NURSES

1. The nurse provides services with respect for human dignity and the uniqueness of the client unrestricted by considerations of social or economic status, personal attributes, or the nature of health problems.
2. The nurse safeguards the client's right to privacy by judiciously protecting information of a confidential nature.
3. The nurse acts to safeguard the client and the public when health care and safety are affected by the incompetent, unethical, or illegal practice of any person.
4. The nurse assumes responsibility and accountability for individual nursing judgments and actions.
5. The nurse maintains competence in nursing.
6. The nurse exercises informed judgment and uses individual competence and qualifications as criteria in seeking consultation, accepting responsibilities, and delegating nursing activities to others.
7. The nurse participates in activities that contribute to the ongoing development of the profession's body of knowledge.
8. The nurse participates in the profession's efforts to implement and improve standards of nursing.
9. The nurse participates in the profession's efforts to establish

and maintain conditions of employment conducive to high-quality nursing care.

10. The nurse participates in the profession's effort to protect the public from misinformation and misrepresentation and to maintain the integrity of nursing.

11. The nurse collaborates with members of the health professions and other citizens in promoting community and national efforts to meet the health needs of the public.

(ANA, 1976. Reprinted with permission.)

In addition to guidelines set by the profession, individual health facilities may provide ethical guidelines for health care professionals. Examples of this are human subjects and hospital ethics committees. These committees review proposed research studies to determine if there are risks to clients and their rights. Nurses are often members of such committees and serve as advocates to protect clients as well as the researcher.

Personal values may conflict with professional values, resulting in a dilemma for the nurse. This common conflict creates situations that require the use of a decision–making process. Nurses are accountable for care given and decisions made relative to client care. They are accountable to the client, significant others, other nurses, health care professionals, society, and themselves. Nurses must provide only such care as is within the scope of their knowledge and skills. Nursing practice must be within a legal and ethical framework. To make decisions regarding client care, the nurse must first be aware of the facts in the situation and gain an understanding of the client's goals and perceptions. The second part of the process of decision–making is an understanding of the nurse's own moral structure and personal values. The ways in which a situation is interpreted depend on this structure and influence the ways in which the facts are processed by the individual. The decision must be based on both processes, with the ultimate goal being the best outcome for the client.

Ethical decisions in nursing also are based on moral principles of the profession. Martin (1980) has identified four moral principles related to nursing. The first is belief in the worth and dignity of the individual and involves client rights, informed consent, and right to self-determination. The second principle is that health care should yield general social good and may involve risks in order to advance health. Professional integrity, which involves faithfulness and commitment, is the third principle. The last principle is the belief in the value and validity of scientific truth and scientific method. All of these principles influence the way a nurse makes decisions about ethical issues, as well as the way others in the profession evaluate the decisions made by peers.

Ethical dilemmas in nursing may be related to client care situations and nursing practice. Ethical dilemmas related to client care situations may involve the nurse in the client advocate element and in assisting the client with decision making. One method that has been presented as a means of resolving this type of ethical problem is collaborative decision–making, in which all professionals involved in a client's health care meet and discuss ethical concerns. The decision reached is then based on several professional and personal values; thus the decision may be more objective, less subject to bias. The National League for Nursing (NLN) has formulated the following document on nursing's role in patient rights, which assists with dilemmas regarding client care.

NURSING'S ROLE IN PATIENTS' RIGHTS

NLN believes the following are patients' rights which nurses have responsibility to uphold:

- People have the right to health care that is accessible and that meets professional standards, regardless of setting.
- Patients have the right to courteous and individualized health care that is equitable, humane and given without discrimination as to race, color, creed, sex, national origin, source of payment, or ethical or political beliefs.
- Patients have the right to information about their diagnosis, prognosis, and treatment—including alternatives to care and risks involved—in terms they and their families can readily understand, so that they can give their informed consent.
- Patients have the legal right to informed participation in all decisions concerning their health care.
- Patients have the right to information about the qualifications, names, and titles of personnel responsible for providing their health care.
- Patients have the right to refuse observation by those not directly involved in their care.
- Patients have the right to privacy during interview, examination, and treatment.
- Patients have the right to privacy in communicating and visiting with persons of their choice.
- Patients have the right to refuse treatments, medications, or participation in research and experimentation, without punitive action being taken against them.

- Patients have the right to coordination and continuity of health care.
- Patients have the right to appropriate instruction or education from health care personnel so that they can achieve an optimal level of wellness and an understanding of their basic health needs.
- Patients have the right to confidentiality of all records (except as otherwise provided for by law or third-party payer contracts) and all communications, written or oral, between patients and health care providers.

(NLN, 1977. Reprinted with permission.)

Nurses are influential in client decision making and must be aware of their own values to avoid misuse of this power over clients. Some other ethical concerns of nurses related to client care situations are behavior control and involuntary hospitalization of psychiatric clients, genetic engineering, reception of donor parts, artificial insemination, autopsy, and euthanasia.

Ethical dilemmas related to nursing practice may include the areas of collective bargaining, hospital policies, nurses' rights, research on clients and nurses, consumer involvement in health care, peer review, and nursing values in conflict with those of other health care professions. Ethical considerations of research include informed consent of persons of all ages, risks to the client versus benefits, methodology, research design, research interventions, and confidentiality and anonymity. For instance, and adult client who agrees to be a subject has a right to determine participation in a research study. Informed consent, freedom from harm, privacy, anonymity, and confidentiality must be considered before involvement of a subject in the study. **Informed consent** refers to a decision for participation after a subject has had instruction on the involvement required, including benefits and potential harm. The subject has the right to refuse participation at any time during the study. Oftentimes the ethical issues are complex and require complex decision making by the researcher regarding application of ethical principles. Any digression from the ethical guidelines must be approached seriously, and reasons for the digression must be validated to others. All research projects must be reviewed by a human subjects committee to ensure that consideration has been given to ethical issues.

It is part of nursing responsibility to actively participate in the formation of policy within various health care organizations where various ethical issues may arise. The area of transplants is a prime example. What guides the decisions regarding the number of times one person can receive an organ when there are persons on a waiting list for these same organs who have not had the opportunity for any transplants? Situations involving a child born with a congenital defect or a child who is being sustained by a ventilator following a car accident are other examples. How long should children in these kinds of situations be sustained by artificial support systems? Who makes the decision regarding removal of the support systems? What are the guidelines for decision-making? Who has what rights in these situations? Nurses, as a part of their professional responsibility, participate in organizational policy and decision–making in these and many other similar ethical situations.

Finally, ethical dilemmas relative to health care and nursing may arise within the larger society. Periodically, for instance, issues are raised related to unlicensed personnel about who is to provide care to clients and what is to be the level of care. This is often an issue seen at a national level. Professional responsibility demands the active participation of nurses who help set policy in such areas.

The promotion of the profession is a third area of possible ethical dilemmas. This may include the issues of baccalaureate entry level for professional nursing, research issues with nurses and clients, sexual discrimination, and autonomy. Curtin (1980) identifies the area of autonomy as the most "pervasive ethical problem; nurses are not free to practice nursing"(p. 27). Traditionally, the practice of nursing has not been recognized as separate from medical and other health care practice areas. This has contributed to the control of nurses by other health care professionals. The traditional role of women has compounded the problem and fostered the nonautonomous, subservient role of nurses. Today, as the consciousness of nurses is raised and increased research and theory development is conducted, nurses are asserting themselves as professionals. Nursing practice presumes accountability for nursing care to meet client care needs. Nurses' values related to the care of clients, professional guidelines, and the more traditional, dependent role of the nurse, with administrators and physicians in control of health care decisions, all may pose ethical dilemmas for the nurse. If payment for services comes from the institution, it may be difficult for the nurse to focus primary concern on the individual and working to satisfy the institution may become the primary concern. Nurses need to realize that they are influential in effecting change in the health care delivery system by using their individual and collective power within an ethical framework. It is important that nurses be able to identify the ethical problem, identify the issues and factors involved, determine who is involved and what part each is to play in the decision making, be aware of the beliefs and values of each involved party, consider the alternatives and the possible consequences of each alternative, identify conflicts, and be able to make a decision.

Throughout the educational process, these and other ethical dilemmas should be studied within the context of the particular nurse–client situation. Faculty and nursing staff act as role models in helping students develop a valid decision-making process. This process is needed to clarify values and arrive at decisions based on an ethical code within a professional value system.

LEGAL CONSIDERATIONS

The legal aspects of health care are closely aligned with ethical concerns. Laws are the enforcement of the "ethical shoulds." Conflicts in the legal system can arise from an ethical problem. Informed consent has already been discussed as it related to a research study, but informed consent is also used in practice settings. It is required before any treatment procedures may be instituted for clients. At times, it may be a legal constraint that generates an ethical problem concerning the amount of information furnished to the client. For instance, legally, the client must be informed of the reason for a procedure; however, the nurse has been directed by the family to withhold information from the client. Thus, the amount of information to be provided raises ethical and legal considerations.

It is essential for nurses to be knowledgeable about the law as it applies to nursing. Accountability and practice, inherent in all professions, form the basis for legal determination. Today, new facets of accountability have come to the foreground because of the public availability of records, emphasis on decision making, evaluation, and demands for consumer rights. In addition, rapid changes in technology—resulting in the use of equipment, new techniques, and procedures that cause changes in health and nursing practice—have contributed to the need for legal decisions not previously encountered. Through modern media the public continues to be informed of trends in health and in specific treatments and their effects, thus contributing to consumerism. Increased technology and specialization have contributed to the depersonalization of health care. Because of fragmentation within the health care system, consumers are more detached from their health care providers than in the past. Thus, they are more likely to seek redress from those providers when things go wrong. Consumer dissatisfaction with care can be expressed through legal channels. Consequently, the legal aspects of health care have become more prominent. Society's formulation of rights related to health care is often reflected in legal terms.

As stated earlier, nurses as professionals are responsible for their own actions. While this responsibility is ethically based on personal and professional values, it is also a legal responsibility grounded in societal needs for health care. The nurse's role in various health care areas and the degree to which the nurse participates have been extended, necessitating knowledge in the legal aspect of nursing. Laws protect the client, ensuring the availability of qualified health care providers and setting standards for practice and monitoring them.

Laws arise out of the need to maintain order in a social system. The more complex the social structure, the more complex the legal system. Laws as well as the professional organization set parameters for nursing practice. It is essential that nurses provide input in the development of laws governing practice and that they monitor issues and related bills affecting nursing and health care. The professional nursing organization employs staff members to assist in these functions. Laws governing nursing practice (nurse practice acts) are discussed below.

Credentialing

Credentialing is a broad term often used to refer to those activities aimed at determining and maintaining specific standards to ensure the safety of the public. One type of credentialing sets minimum standards for governmental licensure and registration. Another type provides a voluntary process for accreditation and certification.

Governmental Licensure and Registration

A license is a legal permit or credential awarded by an agency of the government to persons to engage in a given profession. The purpose of nursing **licensure** is to ensure minimal standards for safe nursing practice and to protect the public from unsafe and incompetent health care practices. Licensure in nursing originated at the turn of the 20th century, when many hospitals were opening their own schools of nursing to provide staff for the hospitals. Many of these nursing programs did not have established standards or a formal curriculum. Students were taught by the apprenticeship method, the length of the programs varied from 6 to 36 months with a focus on service, not education, and the quality of the nurses graduating from these programs could not be monitored (Hamilton, 1996 p. 80). The Nurses' Associated Alumni (now the American Nurses Association) was concerned about the preparation of these graduates and furnished the impetus for states to develop laws governing licensure for nursing practice. In 1902, North Carolina, New York, New Jersey, and Virginia passed permissive laws defining optional standards for nursing practice; by 1909, 20 states had nurse practice laws. In 1938, New York became the first state to make licensure mandatory. Mandatory licensure requires that a person obtain a license to practice nursing by successfully completing an approved program of study and passing the licensure examination (**National Council Licensure Examination-Registered Nurses NCLEX-RN**). This differs from the former permissive licensure, which permitted persons to practice nursing without a license. However, under permissive licensure, an individual could not use the title RN. Permissive laws did not protect the consumer from unqualified care providers; therefore, most states have now adopted mandatory licensure laws.

Registration is a term indicating that basic competency exists or certain qualifications have been met. Registration generates an official register of persons meeting certain criteria and competency. Each state maintains a roster of all nurses who have passed the NCLEX-RN.

Until 1982, the licensure examination, the National Test Pool, had been in use since 1944. Five major areas were tested: medical and surgical nursing, obstetrics, pediatrics, and psychiatric nursing. The **National Council of State Boards of Nursing (NCSBN)** changed the test format in 1982. The title of the examination changed from National State Board Testing Pool (NSBTP) to National Council Licensure Examination (NCLEX). In the changed format, the examination is organized into multiple-choice categories based on client needs and the nursing process. Test items are constructed to examine understanding of knowledge base and locus of decision making. Locus of decision making refers to the relationship of the nurse and the client in determining the state of health of the client in areas amenable to nursing interventions, client-centered goals, and nursing interventions. Questions regarding client needs include: safe and effective care environment (15 percent to 21 percent of the questions), physiological integrity (46 percent to 54 percent of the questions), psychosocial integrity (8 percent to 16 percent of the questions), and health promotion-health maintenance (17 percent to 23 percent of the questions). Questions regarding the nursing process include 17 percent to 23 percent questions in each of the following steps: assessing, analyzing, planning, implementing, and evaluating (NCSBN, 1994).

Beginning in 1994, the NCLEX examination has been administered through **computer-adaptive testing (CAT)**. The CAT consists of multiple-choice questions viewed on a computer screen. The computer program selects questions from a large bank of questions so that different individuals receive equivalent though not identical questions. Each response is evaluated by the computer program before the next question is selected. A slightly harder or easier question is selected according to the previous correct or incorrect response. The computer program is able to ensure that all areas are tested with a balance of easy items to difficult ones. Each question and all possible answers are shown on the screen. Examinees need to press only two computer keys throughout the examination; the space bar moves between possible answers and the enter key is used to make a selection. Unlike the previous paper-and-pencil test format, once an answer has been selected, it is not possible to go back to that item. All candidates answer a minimum of 75 questions and a maximum of 265 questions during the testing period. The maximum length of time for the examination is five hours, but it can be completed in a shorter amount of time, depending on the individual's performance. Rather than a set location and time for the test to be administered to a group of candidates as in the previous protocol, individuals make an appointment at a testing center. The examination is scored by the computer and the individual receives a pass or fail score. The test is designed to test minimal safe practice and not levels of knowledge or practice, so a numerical score is not used. Scores are based on a criterion-referenced standard and there is not a preestablished fixed percentage of passes or failures. Individuals receive their score from the state board of nursing within several weeks after completion of the examination (NCSBN, 1994).

In order to qualify to take the NCLEX-RN, each applicant must have completed a state approved nursing program preparing for registered nursing, pay a fee, and be of good moral character. Each state may also have other particular requirements that must be met before a person qualifies to take the examination. An individual who has been convicted of a felony or who has a record of certain types of misdemeanors may not be permitted to take the state licensing examination without a review.

Graduating from a state-approved school of nursing and passing the registration examination mean that minimal competencies to practice nursing are met. Every state has its own **nurse practice act,** which defines the requirements for licensure, registration, and legal guidelines for practice. These acts protect the nurse's professional practice and legally monitor and control nursing practice. Nurses, individually and in groups, are responsible for familiarizing themselves with the nurse practice acts in the state in which they practice. They are also responsible for providing input for changing and updating the practice acts.

A nurse practice act in each state usually includes statements about a state's board of nursing authority, definition of nursing, scope of practice, requirements for licensure, and it determines legal titles and abbreviations that nurses can use and identifies grounds for disciplinary action. Each act defines the requirements for licensure, registration, and legal guidelines for nursing practice in that particular state.

The nurse practice act in each state is enforced and interpreted by a **board of nursing** established for this purpose. Board composition varies from state to state. Membership may include nurses, consumers, or physicians. Stahl (1974, p. 508) lists the board's responsibilities as:

1. Establish minimal standards for schools of nursing.
2. Survey programs on nursing to determine whether the minimal standards are being met.
3. Place programs meeting the standards on the state approval list.
4. Select, administer, and determine the passing score on the licensing examination.
5. Grant licenses by examination and by interstate endorsement.
6. Renew licenses.
7. Prosecute violators of the law.
8. Revoke or suspend licenses for cause.

See Appendix C for a complete list of the members of the National Council of State Boards of Nursing.

Accreditation

Accreditation is certification of an organization and is a voluntary process that indicates that certain criteria or standards have been met. The NLN (National League for Nursing) is the designated accrediting agency for schools of nursing. (See Chap. 7). The membership in the NLN identifies and votes on the standards and criteria to be met by schools of nursing. Areas that are reviewed include structure and governance, facilities, faculty, students, curriculum, and evaluation. Specific to baccalaureate nursing programs are criteria that focus on critical thinking, therapeutic nursing interventions, and communication.

Certification

Certification is a voluntary, professional form of recognition and professional achievement that validates advanced knowledge and skills of nurses in specific areas of practice. Certification can be obtained through the ANA (American Nurses Association) or through other professional organizations.

The **American Nurses Credentialing Center (ANCC)** was established as a separately incorporated center for the ANA. There are ten boards on certification of the ANCC that develop test items, set passing scores, determine eligibility requirements, and certify all nurses who pass the examination. These boards are:

- Community Health Nursing Practice
- General Nursing Practice
- Maternal-Child Nursing Practice
- Medical-Surgical Nursing Practice
- Psychiatric and Mental Health Nursing Practice
- Primary Care in Adult and Family Health Nursing Practice
- Gerontological Nursing Practice
- Nursing Administration Practice
- Nursing Continuing Education/Staff Development
- Informatics Nursing

Effective in 1998, all generalist examinations will require a baccalaureate or higher degree in nursing. Nurse practitioner and clinical specialist certification requires a master's or higher degree in nursing. Certification is valid for five years, at which time the certification must be renewed (ANCC, 1996).

Certification may also be obtained from other professional nursing and health care organizations. For example, the National Association of Pediatric Nurse Associates/Practitioners (NAPNAP) certifies pediatric nurse practitioners, the Association for Women's Health, Obstetric, and Neonatal Nursing (AWHONN) certifies nurses in the areas of its concern, and the National Association of Orthopedic Nurses (NAON) certifies nurses in the area of orthopedics. Specialty organizations can be contacted to receive more information on specific certification guidelines. A list of specialty organizations can be found in Appendix B.

Law in Nursing Practice

An understanding of the source of **laws** can provide insight into the legal aspects of nursing practice. The source of laws are twofold. The first are **statutory laws,** which come from legislative groups. These laws are rules and regulations based on some social need or a need to maintain social order. State nurse practice acts are an example of statutory law. These acts were written to protect the public from unsafe nursing practice. **Common law** is the second source of law; it often arises from a court ruling on statutory or common law. Criminal law applies to acts that threaten society. **Civil law** is concerned with the protection of individual rights. Violation of a civil law is referred to as a tort, which is failure to act as a reasonably prudent person would have acted in a similar situation. Torts result in monetary loss to compensate for the injury. An example of a tort as applied to health care is **negligence.** Nursing is concerned with health care delivery to individuals and preservation of consumer rights through law (Ellis & Hartley, 1995; Fenner, 1980).

Some of the current legal issues involving health care providers include confidentiality, informed consent, libel, slander, false imprisonment, assault, battery, and negligence.

Examples of legal issues in nursing practice follow.

Case 1. A nurse working in an extended care facility is caring for a stroke patient with left-sided paralysis. The patient is unable to move independently from side to side and is therefore at risk for development of pressure ulcers. Safe, reasonable, and prudent nursing practice would dictate assessing the skin and turning the patient from side to side every 2 hours to prevent a pressure ulcer from developing. Failure to do this could result in **malpractice.**

Case 2. The nurse administers a medication to a client prior to surgery. In this case, the physician prescribed 150 mg. of meperidine (pain medication) intramuscularly to be given to an elderly female client who weighed 100 pounds. After considering the age, weight, and height of the client, the nurse determined that this was not within a safe dosage range for the woman. Legally, the nurse must clarify the order with the physician. If doubt remains and a decision is made on the basis of scientific knowledge, the nurse must relate this to the physician and decline to give the medication.

Nurses as caregivers must meet safe standards of care and perform as "reasonable and prudent" persons. Nursing care is based on the premise of the nurse's being a conscientious, prepared, knowledgeable, and skilled practitioner. Nurses are liable for their actions; therefore, they carry malpractice insurance to protect themselves against **liability** claims. The wisest or best safeguard in nursing practice is for nurses to employ decision making based on nursing process and to ensure that their communication skills are therapeutic when interacting with clients.

LEGAL RESPONSIBILITIES OF THE NURSING STUDENT

Personal Liability

Nursing students are legally responsible for their own actions and can be guilty of malpractice, which is any professional misconduct or negligence. There are legal implications to be considered by students interested in entering nursing. Any individual who has been convicted of a felony is not permitted to take the state licensing examination for nursing practice without review. Students also have legal responsibilities to consider during their nursing education; they cannot perform any function for which they have not received education, and they are accountable for any actions they perform.

Therefore, it is essential for students to know their limitations and seek guidance as needed from their nursing professors. Faculty members provide guidance for students in the use of the decision-making process in determining parameters for safe nursing practice. They are also available during clinical practice times to support students and provide guidelines for specific nursing activities.

Liability Insurance

All nursing professional and students should carry personal and professional liability insurance to provide legal assistance in the event of malpractice. Even though a nurse or nursing student may practice in a reasonable and prudent manner, mistakes can be made. Professional liability insurance can provide legal assistance as well as protect personal assets. Professional liability insurance is available from most state nurses' associations at a reasonable cost for nursing students.

SUMMARY

Ethical considerations of nursing practice were presented. Personal and professional values, moral principles, and ethical dilemmas were related to decision making and accountability in the delivery of nursing care. Legal considerations of nursing practice were presented in terms of credentialing the laws.

Credentialing relates to activities aimed at delivering and maintaining educational competency through accreditation, providing means for voluntary certification, and setting minimum standards for governmental licensure and registration. Ethical and legal ramifications for nursing practice have increased as a result of expanding technology and nursing's broadened scope of practice.

▶ Questions for Discussion

1. What ethical dilemmas that concern nursing practice are you familiar with?
2. What are some of the standards and codes developed to protect consumer rights in nursing care delivery?
3. What protection does the law offer to consumers and the nurse?
4. How do the voluntary and nonvoluntary forms of credentialing differ?
5. What are some legal issues concerning health care?

REFERENCES

American Nurses Association. *Code for Nurses.* Kansas City, MO: ANA; 1976.

American Nurses Credentialing Center. 1996 Certification, Washington, D.C.: ANA; 1996.

Bandman E, Bandman B. *Nursing Ethics Through the Lifespan.* 3rd ed. Norwalk, CT: Appleton & Lange; 1995.

Curtin L. Ethical issues in nursing and nursing education. In: *Ethical Issues in Nursing and Nursing Education.* (NLN publication #16-1822). New York: National League for Nursing; 1980; 19–28.

Czmowski M. Value teaching in nursing education. *Nurs Forum.* 1974; 13:192–206.

Donaldson S, Crowley D. The discipline of nursing. *Nurs Outlook.* 1978; 26:113–120.

Ellis J, Hartley C. *Nursing in Today's World: Challenges, Issues, and Trends.* 5th ed. Philadelphia: Lippincott; 1995.

Fenner K. *Ethics and Law in Nursing: Professional Perspectives.* New York: Van Nostrand; 1980.

Hamilton M. *Realities of contemporary nursing.* 2nd ed. Menlo Park, CA: Addison-Wesley Nursing; 1996.

Martin R. Ethical issues in present-day health care. In: *Ethical Issues in Nursing and Nursing Education* (NLN Publication #16-1822). New York: National League for Nursing; 1980; p 1–17.

National Council of State Boards of Nursing Candidate Bulletin Educational Testing Service. Princeton, NJ; 1994.

Stahl A. State boards of nursing: Legal aspects. *Nurs Clin North Am.* 1974; 9:505.

Thompson J, Thompson H. *Ethics in Nursing.* New York: Macmillan; 1981.

BIBLIOGRAPHY

Benoliel JQ. Ethics in nursing practice and education. *Nurs Outlook.* 1983; 31:210–215.

Besch LB. Informed consent: A patient's right. *Nurs Outlook.* 1979; 27:32–35.

Bullough B. *The Law and the Expanding Nursing Role.* 2nd ed. New York: Appleton-Century-Crofts; 1980.

Evans L, Dienemann J, Dahlert R. University-based nursing research centers: A strategic investment. *Nurs Economics.* 1986; 4:23–30.

Evers S. Nursing Ethics: The central concept of nursing education. *Nurse Educ.* 1984; 9(3):14–18.

Fiesta J. *The Law and Liability, a Guide for Nurses.* New York: Wiley; 1983.

Former M. Abortion ethics. *Nurs Outlook.* 1982; 30:324–240.

Fowler MD. Nursing and social ethics. In: Chaska NL, ed. *The Nursing Profession: Turning Points.* St. Louis: Mosby; 1990. p 24–30.

Fowler MD. Professional associations, ethics, and society. *Oncol Nurs Forum.* 1993; 20 10, Suppl.

Hull R. Responsibility and accountability, analyzed. *Nurs Outlook*. 1981; 23:707–712.

Levine ME. Nursing ethics and the ethical nurse. *Am J Nurs*. 1977; 77:845–847.

National League for Nursing. *National Ethical Issues in Nursing and Nursing Education*. (NLN publication #16-1822) New York: NLN; 1980.

O'Rourke K, Barton S. *Nurse Power: Unions and the Law*. Bowie, MD: Brady; 1981.

Romanell P. Ethics, moral conflicts, and choice. *Am J Nurs*. 1977; 77:850.

Rozovsky LE. Answers to the 15 legal questions nurses usually ask. *Nurs*. 1978; 78:873.

Shannon ML. Nurses in American history. Our first four licensure laws. *Am J Nurs*. 1975; 75:1327–1329.

Sward K. The code for nurses: A guide for ethical nursing practice. *NYS Nurs Assoc*. 1975; 625.

White D, Hamel P. National center for nursing research: How it came to be. *Nurs Econ*. 1986; 4:19–22.

....
....
....
....
....
....

Future Directions in Nursing

Since the first edition of this book, in 1981, many changes have occurred in nursing and in health care. Nursing has grown as a profession and a practice-oriented discipline. Theory development from ongoing research has improved our understanding of health and illness care. Nursing's need for knowledge development and a theoretical basis for practice have necessitated the move toward baccalaureate education as the minimum for entry to professional nursing. Master's-level education has become a necessity for entry to advanced practice and doctoral-level education is needed to continue theory and research development. This is especially true for research in health promotion, outcome measures of nursing interventions in care in the community, and disease prevention

As the health care environment continues to change, issues surrounding the future direction of nursing will come from changes in society as a whole as well as from changes within the profession. Societal shifts from an illness orientation to one of health promotion and wellness care at the community level are central issues for nursing today and in the future. These changes are altering the way health care and nursing care is delivered. Some of the societal influences impacting on nursing are increased health care costs, increased technology, increased aging populations, number of underserved populations, and populations at risk.

Improved technology has proven to be a two-edged sword. The computer age has improved communication and the rapid transmission of information worldwide. Computers are used in all facets of care, from the documentation of care to diagnostic and monitoring procedures. Increased technology has revolutionized health care practices and improved surgical techniques, computerized diagnostic tools have decreased the amount of time persons spend in the hospital.

These advances have also increased the cost of care, increased the need for extended and sub-acute care, decreased the number of occupied hospital beds, caused the number of hospital-based nursing job opportunities to decrease, and drawn attention to alternative care delivery models. In light of in-hospital job opportunity decline, opportunities for nurses to be employed outside of the hospital in community settings have increased. Nurses need to be educated to function in community-based health care. Nursing's focus is caring for the whole person as the center of health care and health care promotion, not just disease cure. Nursing's ability to meet the changes of society will depend on its ability to share a sense of direction for the profession and not be directed by insurance companies, hospitals, or physicians. Nurses pursuing advanced practice opportunities, especially as primary care providers, have dramatically increased over the past few years, making health care more accessible to all populations, especially those in underserved areas. Primary care services are essential to address the high cost of care associated with managing chronic illnesses. Nursing is moving to have full prescriptive authority, third-party reimbursement, and removal of barriers that impede advanced nursing practice. At the same time nurses will be instrumental in cost-containment strategies.

The increased life expectancy and increased number of aging Americans has resulted in the demand for nurses skilled in the care of the elderly with chronic and disabling conditions in nonhospital ambulatory settings. The emphasis on cultural diversity and care for populations at risk must be promoted. Nursing curriculums need to address these issues.

The high cost of hospital care and the increase in health care promotion activities are frequently cited as major trends today. Quality of health care, competition in health care, the increased numbers of uninsured and underinsured individuals, and ethical concerns from changing technology are other societal issues that affect nursing. The consumer movement has increased the awareness and demand for quality care at a reasonable cost. Americans have more opportunity to shop around for health care services, and competition among health care providers has changed the methods of obtaining health care. Managed care programs and alternatives to hospitalization have proliferated. What is health care's price and will consumers be willing to pay the price are questions for the future. The consumer movement has also heightened public awareness of ethical issues. Examples of ethical dilemmas facing Americans are such questions as when to use high-tech interventions and when to terminate advanced life support for a low-birth-weight baby or an adult with a severe head injury. Solutions to these dilemmas are challenges for the nursing profession and the society as a whole.

Nurses are becoming more active in cost management through health promotion activities such as direct client intervention, health policy, and health legislation. Nurses can significantly increase health promoting activities and decrease health care costs through health education programs, early crisis intervention, and assessment of ineffective health practices. Consumers will need the education to be self-directed in their care.

Nursing as a community-based, culturally aware discipline and profession is essential to the promotion of health and well-being in our changing society. Nurses must autonomously direct educational preparation of nurses; engage in nursing research and theory development; educate consumers in effective health care practices; and influence health care legislation.

Even with all the changes occurring around us, it is an exciting time to be in nursing. This book was designed to provide a foundation for nursing students to understand nursing as a profession and a discipline and nursing's relationship with health care. We hope that your experiences in nursing are positive and rewarding

BIBLIOGRAPHY

Knollmueller R. Thinking about tomorrow for nursing: Changes and challenges. *J Continuing Edu Nurs.* 1994; 25(5):196–201.

Meleis A. Directions for nursing theory development in the 21st century. *Nurs Sci Q.* 1992; 5(3):112–117.

Glossary

AACN. American Association of Colleges of Nursing.

Abstract for Action. See Lysaught Report.

Accountability. Responsibility for one's own actions.

Accreditation. Voluntary process of evaluation and credentialing that shows preset standards and criteria have been met.

Acute. Short-term, self-limiting illness that, unlike chronic illness, is treated and cured.

Advanced practice nurse (APN). A broad term for nurses who have completed educational preparation at the graduate level to acquire the needed knowledge and practice experiences for specialization.

Affective. Related to the emotions and attitudes.

AHCPR. Agency for Health Care Policy and Research. Established in 1989 to enhance the quality, appropriateness, and effectiveness of health care services and access to these services.

Altruism. Giving for the benefit of others rather than for self-gain.

Ambulatory care. Health services provided to persons outside the hospital setting on an outpatient basis.

Ambulatory clinic. Area of health care where clients walk in, receive treatment, and return home.

American Nurses Association (ANA). Professional nurses' organization formed to establish and control policies and activities of nursing practice. Establishes standards of practice and code of ethics. Promotes professional and education advancement.

American Nurses Association Position Paper. Statement made by the professional nursing organization in 1965 concerning nursing education and entry levels into practice.

Analysis. A process involving the interpreting and making of a judgment regarding related data.

ANCC. The American Nurses Credentialing Center, established as a separately incorporated center for the ANA. Ten boards on certification of the ANCC develop test items, set passing scores, determine eligibility requirements, and certify all nurses who pass the examination.

Androgogy. Principles of adult education as proposed by Knowles.

Apprentice. One who agrees to work in return for instruction.

Assessment. Collection and analysis of data.

Associate Degree. Title conferred after completion of a particular course of study, generally for 2 years, in a college setting.

Autonomy. Establishing and controlling own policies and activities; independence in performance of functions and actions; taking individual responsibility.

Auxiliary personnel. Personnel on the nursing team without professional education in nursing.

Baccalaureate degree. Degree conferred after completion of a 4-year course of study in a particular content area, in a college or university setting.

Becoming. Dynamic view of the person in "search of self" and of highest potential.

Board of nursing. A board established in each state to enforce and interpret the state's nurse practice act. Board composition varies from state to state. Membership may include nurses, consumers, or physicians.

Boundary. External limits.

Brown Report (*Nursing for the Future*). Esther Lucille Brown's 1948 report on nursing service and nursing education.

Capitation. Health care financed by a prepaid fee for service.

Caregiver. One who renders physical, psychosocial, and spiritual care.

Case management. Type of health care delivery where a case manager follows a client through an entire episode of care.

Case-method research. Form of research involving analysis for causation and interrelationship of variables.

CAT. The National Council Licensure Examination (NCLEX) is administered through computer-adaptive testing (CAT), which consists of multiple choice questions viewed on a computer screen. The computer program selects questions from a large bank of questions so that individuals receive equivalent though not identical questions.

CDC. Centers for Disease Control and Prevention. Agency responsible for prevention of communicable disease and promotion of the health of the entire community.

Certification. Form of credentialing where voluntary recognition is given for knowledge and skills of nurses in specific areas of practice.

Change. Process by which a person, situation, or thing becomes different.

Change agent. Planner of change using a planned, collaborative, systematic method.

Chronic. Pertaining to long-term illness, usually treated but not cured.

Civil law. Laws for the protection of individual rights.

Client advocate. One who defends and protects client rights, acts on behalf of client.

Clinic. Acute care or rehabilitation center for ambulatory clients.

Clinical specialist. Nurse with advanced preparation, usually a master's degree, in a specialty area. Able to provide advanced levels of client care.

Code of ethics. Code, established by a professional organization, that provides ethical guidelines for professional conduct and forms a foundation for evaluating professional performance by the public and within the profession.

Cognitive domain. Mental process, acquisition of knowledge, use of judgment, memory, understanding, and reasoning.

Collaborator. One who works with others to meet a need or goal that cannot be met by individuals alone.

Common law. Source of law arising from a court ruling on statutory law.

Community college. A local college designed to meet the educational needs of the people of a particular geographic location and often offering 2-year associate degree programs.

Concept. Idea; a label, or naming of an object.

Conceptual model. Structure comprising concepts or abstract ideas that provide a way of viewing a particular area or phenomenon of interest.

Consultant. One who exchanges views among health care providers to clarify goals and plans.

Consumer. One who utilizes services or goods.

Continuum. Sequence; items in an ongoing and ordered sequence.

Coordinator. One who arranges in proper order or brings into harmony.

Counselor. One who advises by identifying dysfunctional patterns of interaction and planning for methods of establishing functional patterns.

Credentialing. Activities aimed at determining and maintaining educational competency through accreditation, providing means for voluntary certification and setting minimum standards by governmental licensure and registration.

Critical thinking. Process as a basis for patient nursing care decisions as well as understanding and functioning within the health care delivery system and the profession of nursing.

Culture. Characteristics or behaviors of a particular group or society that distinguish it from other groups or societies.

Data. Factual information. Data are both subjective and objective. Data are collected by observation, interview, or interaction.

Dentist. One who has been educated to diagnose and treat oral disorders.

Design. Method by which the research is to be conducted, depending on problem and type of research being done; specifies population sample to be used and method for collecting data.

Development theory. Theory that describes human growth in terms of stages or as changes occurring in smooth transitions.

Diagnosis-related group (DRG). Classification for reimbursement for health care services in acute care settings.

Dietitian. Person educated in the study of nutrition and the application of its principles.

Dilemma. Quandary; problem without solution; predicament.

Diploma. Certification presented to a person after completion of a particular course of study.

Director of nursing. Top-level management position responsible for an entire nursing service department.

Discipline. A body of knowledge that is often expressed in practice and is continually changed and expanded through research.

Doctoral education. Advanced preparation in research and theory development.

Doctorate. Degree conferred after completion of advanced studies in a university setting, preceded by a master's degree.

Dunn, Halbert. Physician who proposed a dynamic view of health on a continuum from wellness to illness.

Educator. One who promotes knowledge through established instructional processes.

Environment. Internal and external conditions involving an open exchange of energy.

Ethics. Principles behind the morals of society.

Ethnographical research. Research aimed at defining and analyzing the life patterns of the people of a culture within their familiar environment.

Ethnoscience. A process or a systematic way of studying from within a culture that particular culture's perceptions of its own universe.

Evaluation. Method of determining if nursing interventions are effective.

Existentialism. Philosophical view in which an individual's uniqueness, values and meaning, self-direction, and self-fulfillment are emphasized.

Experimental research. Type of research where the experiment is controlled and at least one causative factor is manipulated.

Ex-post-facto research. Type of research where data are collected after the event has occurred; it is not controlled and therefore cannot be manipulated.

External factors. Those aspects operating from outside a situation or individual.

Feedback. Information given back to a system.

Field study research. Research conducted outside the laboratory.

Formative evaluation. Evaluation done during the development of project or program.

Functional nursing. Organization and distribution of tasks to facilitate efficient use of time and energy.

Gatekeeper. Primary provider who makes the decisions on referrals to other specialists.

General staff duty. Entry-level position for nurses in the hospital bureaucracy; responsibility for direct client care.

Goal setting. Determination of the questions to be answered in a research project; determination of specific factors; relationships to be studied and appropriate statistical analysis of data (hypothesis).

Goldmark Report. A 1923 study of nursing education (*Nursing and Nursing Education in the United States*); recommended nursing programs be independent of hospitals and that high school graduation be a minimum requirement for entry into programs.

Graduate education. Education beyond the baccalaureate degree; includes master's and doctor's level education.

Grounded theory. Research studies data grounded in fact.

Head nurse. Coordinator of all client care on a specified nursing unit.

Health. Sense of physical, psychological, spiritual, and social well-being; description is dependent on a person's perception.

Health care delivery system. Organization of services to provide for the health of members within a society.

Health promotion. Refers to maintaining and enhancing well-being.

Health screening. Examination aimed at early detection and identification of health problems.

Health care administrator. Person educated in and responsible for the management of a health care agency or organization.

Historical research. Type of research involving interpretations of past events in relation to current and future events.

HMO. Health maintenance organization. Type of managed care organization.

Holistic. Theory describing the interrelatedness of parts to the whole.

Homeostasis. Relative state of balance or equilibrium of the parts in relation to the whole; steady state.

Hospice. Supportive therapy for terminally ill clients and their families.

Hypothesis. Declarative statement to be addressed in a research project.

Infection surveillance nurse. Nurse involved with coordination and education of personnel in recognizing and reporting communicable diseases.

Informal health care. Health care outside the orthodox health care organizations, consisting of cultural and folk health beliefs and systems.

Informed consent. Legal concern involving voluntary consent (agreement) to treatment, where the client is the decision maker and may refuse any aspect of treatment or refuse to participate at any time.

Integrated delivery systems (IDS). An entire continuum of care under one system with the focus on primary care to provide more cost-effective care. A fully operational system uses hospitals, clinics, physicians, nurses, subacute care, home health care, pharmacy, and durable medical goods, covering a broad geographic area.

Internal factors. Those aspects operating from within a situation or individual.

International Council of Nurses (ICN). International nursing organization, of which the American Nurses Association is a member.

Interpersonal process. Goal-directed, purposeful, therapeutic process.

Interpersonal theory. Theory in which individual as a social being in interaction with others is the focus.

Intervention. Planned nursing actions to meet stated goals.

JCAHCO. Joint Commission for Accreditation of Health Care Organizations. Accredits hospitals and nursing services for the purpose of documenting "quality" care.

Kluckhohn, Clyde. Anthropologist who described three facets believed to characterize humans.

Laws. Enforcement of ethics; means of maintaining order of a social structure.

Levels of prevention. Three types of health care consisting of prevention, early diagnosis and treatment, and rehabilitation

Liability. Legal term for a person's responsibility and accountability for wrongful acts through financial compensation.

Licensed practical nurse (LPN). One who has completed an educational program in nursing, generally 1 year in length, and who has passed a state licensing examination.

Licensure. Legal permit serving as a means to protect the public from unsafe and incompetent health care delivery.

Literature review. Step in formal research project that involves reading of literature concerning the variables of the project; includes previous studies conducted and significant findings; and validates need for the project.

Lysaught Report (*Abstract for Action*). 1970 report for the National Commission for the Study of Nursing and Nursing Education.

Malpractice. Legal term for form of negligence where wrongdoing or injudicious treatment resulted in an injury; may be due to misconduct, lack of skill, or failure to act (omission).

Managed care. Managed health care organizations plan health care to control costs effectively. Consumers who belong to a managed care system select a primary health care provider (e.g., family practioner, pediatrician, nurse practioner) under the managed system. This primary provider is the "gatekeeper" and makes the decisions on referrals to other specialists.

Maslow, Abraham. Developed a hierarchy, or levels, of basic human needs in which lower needs must be met before higher needs can be fulfilled.

Master's degree. Title conferred on completion of specialized studies in a university setting beyond the baccalaureate degree.

Medicaid. State and federal program to finance health care for those unable to afford such care.

Medicare. Federally funded program to provide health care, especially to the aged population

Montag, Mildred. Developed concept of associate degree nursing in the early 1950s.

Morals. Societal determination of what "ought" to be done or that "should" be done by members of a society.

NCLEX. National Council Licensure Examination.

NCSBON. National Council of State Boards of Nursing.

National League for Nursing (NLN). Organization formed to assist in the maintenance of the goals and purposes of professional nursing. Membership comprises nurses and other interested persons. A major service is accreditation of nursing schools.

National Student Nurses' Association (NSNA). Professional nursing organization for nursing students.

Needs theory. Theory that focuses on human needs, which appear to be common to the motivations and strivings of individuals to direct behavior toward goal attainment.

Negligence. Legal term used when a person fails to do what a reasonable, prudent person with the same skill or knowledge base would do.

NIC. The Nursing Interventions Classification, created in the early 1990s to help practitioners document their care; help with standardizing language (nomenclature) of nursing treatments; provide a linkage between nursing diagnosis, treatments, and outcomes; expand nursing knowledge; develop information systems, teach decision making to students; determine cost of services provided by nurses; and to articulate with other health care providers.

Nightingale, Florence. Often identified as the founder of modern nursing.

NINR. The National Institute for Nursing Research, a public agency that is part of the National Institutes of Health. Purpose is to award research grants related to patient care, promotion of health, and prevention of disease.

North American Nursing Diagnosis Association (NANDA). Group of nurses whose purpose is to develop nursing diagnoses and classifications.

Nurse administrator. Functions in a variety of settings where nursing management is needed; ensures professional goals are maintained and the atmosphere is conducive to implementing the nursing role.

Nurse anesthetist. Registered nurse educated beyond the baccalaureate degree to administer anesthesia.

Nurse consultant. Registered nurse, usually with a master's degree, who consults with other health care providers.

Nurse educator. Nurse who teaches nursing in a formalized education setting.

Nurse midwife. Provides prenatal, intrapartum, and postpartum care to expectant families.

Nurse practice act. Legal practice act defining or describing the minimum skill and knowledge level needed to practice nursing; protects the public from incompetent nurses.

Nurse practitioner. Registered nurse with advanced educational preparation in health assessment skills; used primarily in ambulatory settings, with a variety of clients and age groups. Assessment includes determining physical and psychosocial health status of patients through history and physical examinations, and evaluating and interpreting findings in order to plan and carry out interventions. Practice in many areas such as pediatrics, family health, adult, geriatrics, community health, and mental health.

Nurse researcher. One who advances theory development through research.

Nursing. Profession and discipline based on the concepts of person, health, and environment with the components of theory, practice, and research; involved with individuals or groups in health maintenance and curative and rehabilitation aspects of health.

Nursing care plan. Communication (oral or written) system relating specific planned nursing interventions; outline of plans for client care.

Nursing center. Nurse managed centers or nursing centers, which render primary care.

Nursing diagnosis. Presents health status to be addressed by nursing intervention; statement of client's unmet needs or health status.

Nursing history. A component of the assessment phase of nursing process involving the collection of data about that aspect of a client's health status amenable to nursing care.

Nursing process. A systematic method of approaching client care, based on a problem-solving method.

Nursing team. Group of nursing personnel to provide care to clients and groups of clients.

Objective data. Factual information obtained by assessment that involves the senses.

Occupational health nurses. Nurses employed in industry and business to provide health care to employees.

Occupational therapy. Planned activity aimed at the rehabilitative aspects of health, including skills necessary for activities of daily living.

Official agency. Tax-supported government agency.

Outcome. Results expected from evaluation or research process, end behaviors.

Paradigm. Model, pattern, or world view.

Pastoral care. Health services related to the spiritual and religious aspects of client care.

Patient's Bill of Rights. Statement of beliefs regarding rights of clients.

Person. Unique, changing, continuous flow of energy with unique needs, ideas, dreams, and goals.

Phenomenon. Occurrence of happening; an observable manifestation, need, or condition.

Phenomenological. Relating to the lived human experience.

Philosophy. Beliefs of a person or group of persons; reveals underlying values and attitudes regarding an area.

Physical therapy. Treatment of ailments by mechanical manipulation of body parts and application of heat or cold.

Physician. Person prepared and licensed to diagnose and treat illness.

PPO. Preferred provider organizations, type of managed care organizations. The network of health care providers agree to deliver services to enrollees at a predetermined fee.

Postmodernism. Represents the end of the western mindset with the dominance of one way of viewing reality or one world view.

Practice. Nursing theory applied in the clinical setting for actual or potential health problems.

Prenatal. Prior to the birth of a child.

Primary health care. Person's first contact with the health care delivery system.

Primary nursing. Nursing care centered around 24-hour responsibility for client care.

Private practice. Situation where nurses practice independent of other professions or organizations

Problem statement. Step in research project involving identification of the problem to be studied and stating it in clear, concise terminology.

Process evaluation. Evaluation conducted during the planning and implementation phases of a project.

Product evaluation. Evaluation conducted at the completion of a project.

Profession. Group of qualified persons engaged in a specific area or occupation.

Professional. One who is competent in a specified area or occupation.

Professional culture. Term related to socialization derived from interaction of students, faculty, and other health care professionals.

Proprietary. Profit-making.

Propositions. Statements linking concepts.

Psychomotor. Skills requiring knowledge and manual dexterity.

Qualitative research. Descriptive, inductive investigation of an area of concern without the use of numbering or counting.

Quality assurance. Organizational structure for evaluation of client care services. In nursing, it involves (1) establishing written care plan; (2) nursing rounds; (3) obtaining client feedback; (4) documentation; and (5) nursing audit.

Quantitative research. Objective, deductive methodology that enables the investigator to count or number the phenomena of interest in order to apply statistical tests to the data.

Registered nurse (RN). A person educated in a college or hospital setting and licensed to practice professional nursing at all levels of health care.

Registration. Process of mandatory credentialing for practice in a specific area, used to demonstrate competency or the attainment of certain qualifications.

Rehabilitation. Health services aimed at restoring an individual to optimal health; focus on physical, psychosocial, and spiritual aspects.

Reliability. Applies to measurement methods used in research studies; the accuracy and consistency of a method.

Report of Committee on the Training of Nurses. AMA study on the training of nurses, headed by Dr. Samuel Gross in 1869.

Research. Systematic approach to the development of knowledge and testing or validation of theory.

Resource Utilization Group (RUG). Classification for reimbursement for health care services with extended care centers.

Respiratory therapy. Treatment related to pulmonary dysfunctions and associated needs.

Role. Position with standard or expected behaviors.

Role development. Personal process of learning and integrating the behaviors of a particular position.

Secondary health care. Cure and restoration.

Self-actualization. Attaining one's highest potential; Maslow's highest need.

Self-care. The practice of being able to care for oneself; involves a healthy lifestyle.

Sigma Theta Tau (STT). International honorary nursing organization with focus on scholarship and research in nursing.

Significant others. Persons who are important to the client; may include family members or friends.

Socialization. The process of becoming a participant in the activities and ways of a particular social group.

Social Policy Statement (ANA). Official statement of the American Nurses' Association concerning the nature and scope of nursing (1980).

Social work. Services aimed at providing social assistance to clients and significant others.

Society. Group of persons with established patterns of relating and socialization.

Staff development. Identifying learning needs of nursing team members, instituting in-service programs for review of skills, and presenting new equipment and policies.

Staff nurse. Entry-level nursing position in hospital settings.

Standards of practice. Measurement scale or model of behaviors and concepts necessary for the provision of quality client care.

Statutory law. Laws that come from legislative groups. These laws are rules and regulations based on some social need or a need to maintain social order.

Stress. Positive or negative psychological and physical response to perceived threats or demands.

Structure evaluation. Refers to obtaining feedback on resources in the environment.

Subject identification. Part of research design that involves identification of means to obtain a study sample that is representative of a population.

Subjective data. Information obtained directly from the client through interviews; what the client thinks or experiences that cannot be seen by others.

Subsystem. Component parts within the system.

Summative evaluation. Evaluation conducted at the completion or end of a project.

Supervisor. Administrator responsible for several nursing units.

Suprasystem. Components outside the system.

Surgeon General's Report (*Toward Quality in Nursing*). A 1963 report identifying the need for nursing schools, areas of society not represented in nursing, and need for research in nursing.

Survey research. Type of research involving the use of questionnaires, polls, etc., to collect data.

System. Unit or element of a larger whole that can be identified as having its own boundaries and functioning and that is interrelated with other systems.

Systems theory. Theory that focuses on the interaction of individuals and their environment and interaction of parts.

Team nursing. Nursing care involving one nurse directing groups of nurses with diversified preparation in nursing care of clients.

Tertiary health care. Specialized and sophisticated care.

Theorist. One who writes or develops a theory.

Theory. Knowledge organized systematically to explain phenomena.

Traditional role. Functions customarily attributed to a particular occupation.

Traditional setting. Area of practice usually associated with nursing.

Transition theory. Theory of life transition as a process that bridges the disruption of reality to a newly constructed reality.

UAP. Unlicensed assistive personnel; are "nurse extenders" and are recruited and trained "on the job" as support personnel to the professional staff.

Unit manager. Person in charge (usually a nurse) of a hospital nursing unit.

Validity. In research methodology, assurance that an instrument measures what the researcher is looking for or what the researcher wants it to measure.

Values. Beliefs held about the worth, truth, and desirability of an idea, object, or behavior; guidelines for personal behavior derived from the individual's life experience, the interpretations of these experiences, and the experiences of others.

Variable. What is to be studied in a research project; a symbol assigned numbers or values for study. Example: In a problem concerning sleeping medications and back rubs for clients, the variables are sleeping medications and back rubs, the elements or constructs to be examined and defined.

Voluntary organization. Nonprofit organization for delivery of health care services supplemented by individuals, gifts, and third-party payments.

von Bertalanffy, Ludwig. Scientist often credited with developing the general systems theory.

Wellness centers. Health-promotion facility; found in a variety of settings, such as industry or local community centers. Health care services usually focus on health promotion and self-care.

World view. Paradigm.

State Nurses Associations

Alabama State Nurses' Association
360 North Hill Street
Montgomery, Alabama 36104-3658

Alaska Nurses Association
237 East Third Avenue
Anchorage, Alaska 99501

American Nurses Association
600 Maryland Avenue S.W., Suite 100
West
Washington, D.C. 20024-2571

Arizona Nurses Association
1850 E. Southern Avenue,
Suite 1
Tempe, Arizona 85282-5832

Arkansas Nurses Association
117 South Cedar Street
Little Rock, Arkansas 72205

California Nurses Association
P.O. Box 225
3010 Wilshire Boulevard
Los Angeles, California 90010

Colorado Nurses Association
5453 East Evans Place
Denver, Colorado 80222

Connecticut Nurses Association
Meritech Business Park
377 Research Parkway, Suite 2D
Meriden, Connecticut 06450

Delaware Nurses Association
2634 Capitol Trail, Suite A
Newark, Delaware 19711

**District of Columbia Nurses
Association, Inc.**
5100 Wisconsin Avenue N.W.,
Suite 306
Washington, D.C. 20016

Florida Nurses Association
P.O. Box 536985
Orlando, Florida 32853-6985

Georgia Nurses Association
1362 West Peachtree Street N.W.
Atlanta, Georgia 30309

Guam Nurses Association
P.O. Box CC
Agana, Guam 96910

Hawaii Nurses Association
677 Ala Moana Boulevard, Suite 307
Honolulu, Hawai 96813

Idaho Nurses Association
200 North 4th Street, Suite 20
Boise, Idaho 83702-6001

Illinois Nurses Association
300 South Wacker, Suite 2200
Chicago, Illinois 60606

Indiana State Nurses Association
2915 North High School Road
Indianapolis, Indiana 46224

Iowa Nurses Association
1501 42nd Street, Suite 471
West Des Moines, Iowa 50266

Kansas State Nurses Association
700 S.W. Jackson, Suite 601
Topeka, Kansas 66603

Kentucky Nurses Association
1400 South First Street, P.O. Box 2616
Louisville, Kentucky 40201

Louisiana State Nurses Association
712 Transcontinental Drive
Metairie, Louisiana 70001

Maine State Nurses Association
P.O. Box 2240
295 Water Street
Augusta, Maine 04330-2240

Maryland Nurses Association
849 International Drive
Airport Square 21, Suite 255
Linthicum, Maryland 21090

Massachusetts Nurses Association
340 Turnpike Street
Canton, Massachusetts 02021

Michigan Nurses Association
2310 Jolly Oak Road
Okemos, Michigan 48864-4599

Minnesota Nurses Association
1295 Bandana Boulevard North,
    Suite 140
St. Paul, Minnesota 55108-5115

Mississippi Nurses Association
135 Bounds Street, Suite 100
Jackson, Mississippi, 39206

Missouri Nurses Association
7904 Bubba Lane, Box 105228
Jefferson City, Missouri 65110

Montana Nurses Association
104 Broadway, Suite G-2
P.O. Box 5718
Helena, Montana 59601

Nebraska Nurses Association
1430 South Street, Suite 202
Lincoln, Nebraska 68502-2446

Nevada Nurses Association
3660 Baker Lane, Suite 104
Reno, Nevada 09509

New Hampshire Nurses Association
48 West Street
Concord, New Hampshire
    03301-3595

New Jersey State Nurses Association
320 West State Street
Trenton, New Jersey 08618-5780

New Mexico Nurses Association
909 Virginia N.E., Suite 101
Albuquerque, New Mexico 87708

New York State Nurses Association
46 Correll Road
Latham, New York 12110

North Carolina Nurses Association
103 Enterprise Street
P.O. Box 12025
Raleigh, North Carolina 27605

North Dakota Nurses Association
549 Airport Road
Bismarck, North Dakota 58504-6107

Ohio Nurses Association
4000 East Main Street
Columbus, Ohio 43213-2983

Oklahoma Nurses Association
6414 North Santa Fe, Suite A
Oklahoma City, Oklahoma 73116

Oregon Nurses Association
9600 S.W. Oak, Suite 550
Portland, Oregon 97223

Pennsylvania Nurses Association
P.O. Box 68525
2578 Interstate Drive
Harrisburg, Pennsylvania 17106-8525

**Rhode Island State Nurses
Association**
550 S. Water Street, Unit 540B
Providence, Rhode Island 02903-4344

**South Carolina Nurses
Association**
1821 Gadsden Street
Columbia, South Carolina 29201

South Dakota Nurses Association
1505 South Minnesota Avenue, Suite 3
Sioux Falls, South Dakota 57105

Tennessee Nurses Association
545 Mainstream Drive, Suite 405
Nashville, Tennessee 37228-1201

Texas Nurses Association
7600 Burnet Road, Suite 440
Austin, Texas 78757-1292

Utah Nurses Association
455 East 400 South, Suite 402
Salt Lake City, Utah 84111

Vermont State Nurses Association
26 Champlain Mill
Winooski, Vermont 05404-2230

**Virgin Islands State Nurses
Association**
P.O. Box 583
Christiansted, St. Croix
U.S. Virgin Islands 00821

Virginia Nurses Association
7113 Three Chopt Road, Suite 204
Richmond, Virginia 23226

Washington State Nurses Association
2505 Second Avenue, Suite 500
Seattle, Washington 98121

West Virginia Nurses Association
2003 Quarrier Street
Charleston, West Virginia 25311-4911

Wisconsin Nurses Association
6117 Monoma Drive
Madison, Wisconsin 53716

Wyoming Nurses Association
Majestic Building, Room 305
1603 Capitol Avenue
Cheyenne, Wyoming 82001

Nursing Specialty Organizations

Academy of Medical-Surgical Nurses
East Holly Avenue, Box 56
Pitman, New Jersey 08071-0056

American Academy of Ambulatory
Care Nursing
East Holly Avenue, Box 56
Pitman, New Jersey 08071-0056

American Academy of Nurse
Practitioners
Capitol Station, LBJ Building
P.O. Box 12846
Austin, Texas 78711

The American Assembly for Men
in Nursing
P.O. Box 31753
Independence, Ohio 44131

American Association of Colleges
of Nursing
One Dupont Circle, Suite 530
Washington, D.C. 20036

American Association of
Critical-Care Nurses
101 Columbia
Aliso Viejo, California 92656-1491

American Association for the History
of Nursing, Inc.
P.O. Box 90803
Washington, D.C. 20090-0803

American Association of Legal Nurse
Consultants
500 N. Michigan Avenue, Suite 1400
Chicago, Illinois 60611

American Association
of Neuroscience Nurses
224 N. Des Plaines, Suite 601
Chicago, Illinois 60661

American Association of Nurse
Anesthetists
222 South Prospect Avenue
Park Ridge, Illinois 60068-4001

The American Association of Nurse
Attorneys (TAANA)
720 Light Street
Baltimore, Maryland 21230

American Association of
Occupational Health Nurses
50 Lenox Pointe
Atlanta, Georgia 30324

American Association of Office Nurses
109 Kinderkamack Road
Monvale, New Jersey 07645

American Association of Spinal Cord Injury Nurses
75-20 Astoria Boulevard
Jackson Heights, New York 11370-1177

American College of Nurse-Midwives
818 Connecticut Avenue, N.W., Suite 900
Washington, D.C. 20006

American Holistic Nurses' Association
4101 Lake Boone Trail, Suite 201
Raleigh, North Carolina 27607

American Nephrology Nurses' Association
East Holly Avenue, Box 56
Pitman, New Jersey 08071-0056

American Nurses Association
600 Maryland Avenue, S.W., Suite 100 West
Washington, D.C. 20024-2571

American Nurses Foundation
600 Maryland Avenue S.W., Suite 100 West
Washington, D.C. 20024

American Organization of Nurse Executives (AONE)
840 N. Lake Shore Drive
Chicago, Illinois 60611

American Psychiatric Nurses' Association
6900 Grove Road
Thorofare, New Jersey 08086

American Society for Long-Term Care Nurses
60 Lonely Cottage Drive
Upper Black Eddy, Pennsylvania 18972-9313

American Society of Ophthalmic Registered Nurses
P.O. Box 193030
San Francisco, California 94119

American Society of Pain Management Nurses
11512 Allecingie Parkway
Richmond, Virginia 23235

American Society of Post Anesthesia Nursing
11512 Allecingie Parkway
Richmond, Virginia 23235

Association of Child and Adolescent Psychiatry
1211 Locust Street
Philadelphia, Pennsylvania 19107

Association of Community Health Nursing Educators
407 North Park Avenue
Indianapolis, Indiana 46202

Association of Nurses in AIDS Care
704 Stonyhill Road, Suite 106
Yardley, Pennsylvania 19067

Association of Operating Room Nurses
2170 S. Parker Road, Suite 300
Denver, Colorado 80231-5711

Association of Pediatric Oncology Nurses
11512 Allecingie Parkway
Richmond, Virginia 23235

Association for Professionals in Control and Epidemiology
1016 16th Street N.W.
Washington, D.C. 20036

Association of Rehabilitation Nurses
5700 Old Orchard Road
Skokie, Illinois 60077

Association of Womens Health, Obstetric, and Neonatal Nurses (AWHONN)

14th Street N.W., Suite 600
Washington, D.C. 20005

Dermatology Nurses Association
East Holly Avenue, Box 56
Pitman, New Jersey 08071-0056

**Developmental Disabilities Nurses
Association**
1720 Willow Creek Circle, Suite 515
Eugene, Oregon 97402

**Drug and Alcohol Nursing
Association, Inc.**
660 Lonely Cottage Drive
Upper Black Eddy, Pennsylvania
18972-9313

Emergency Nurses Association
216 Higgins Road
Park Ridge, Illinois 60068

**Federation of Nurses and Health
Professionals**
555 New Jersey Ave N.W.
Washington, D.C. 20001

Frontier Nursing Service
Wendover, Kentucky 41775

**Midwest Nursing Research Society
(MNRS)**
4700 W. Lake Ave.
Glenview, Illinois 60025-1485

**The National Alliance of Nurse
Practitioners**
325 Pennsylvania Ave S.E.
Washington, D.C. 20003-1100

**National Association of Directors
of Nursing Administrators in
Long-Term Care**
10999 Reed Hartman Highway,
Suite 229
Cincinnati, Ohio 45242

**National Association of Neonatal
Nurses**
1304 Southpoint Boulevard, Suite 280
Petaluma, California 94954-6859

**National Association of Nurse
Practitioners in Reproductive
Health (NANPRH)**
2401 Pennsylvania Avenue N.W.,
Suite 350
Washington, D.C. 20037-1718

**National Association of Orthopedic
Nurses**
East Holly Avenue, Box 56
Pittman, New Jersey 08071-7463

**National Association of Pediatric
Nurse Practitioners**
1101 Kings Highway North, Suite 206
Cherry Hill, New Jersey 08034

**National Association of School
Nurses, Inc.**
P.O. Box 1300
Scarborough, Maine 04074-1300

**National Black Nurses Association,
Inc.**
1012 10th Street N.W.
Washington, D.C. 20001

**National Center for Education
in Maternal and Child Health**
2000 15th Street N, Suite 701
Arlington, Virginia 22201-2617

**National Consortium of Chemical
Dependency Nurses**
1720 Willow Creek Circle, Suite 519
Eugene, Oregon 97402

**National Council of State Boards
of Nursing, Inc.**
676 N. St. Clair, Suite 550
Chicago, Illinois 60611-2921

**National Federation for Specialty
Nursing Organizations**
East Holly Avenue, Box 56
Pitman, New Jersey 08071-0056

National Flight Nurses Association
6900 Grove Road
Thorofare, New Jersey 08086

National Gerontological Nursing
  Association
7250 Parkway Drive, Suite 510
Hanover, Maryland 21076

National League for Nursing
350 Hudson Street
New York, New York 10014

National Nurses in Business
  Association
1000 Burnett Avenue, Suite 450
Concord, California 94520

National Organization for Associate
  Degree Nursing
1730 N. Lynn Street, Suite 502
Arlington, Virginia 22209-2004

National Nurses Society
  on Addictions
4101 Lake Boone Trail, Suite 201
Raleigh, North Carolina 27607

National Nursing Staff Development
  Organization
437 Twin Bay Drive
Pensacola, Florida 32534-1350

National Student Nurses'
  Association
555 W. 57th Street, Suite 1327
New York, New York 10019

North American Nursing Diagnosis
  Association
1211 Locust Street
Philadelphia, Pennsylvania 19107

Nurses Christian Fellowship
6400 Schroeder Road, P.O. Box 7895
Madison, Wisconsin 53707-7895

Nurses for the Environment
P.O. Box 22118
Juneau, Alaska 99802-2118

Nurses Environmental Health
  Watch
181 Marshall Street
Duxbury, Massachusetts 03443

Nurse Healers Professional Associates
175 5th Avenue, Suite 2755
New York, New York 10001

Nurses Organization of Veterans
  Affairs
1726 M Street N.W., Suite 1101
Washington, D.C. 20036

Nursing Archives
Boston University, Mugar Memorial
771 Commonwealth Avenue
Boston, Massachusetts 02215

Nursing Network on Violence
  Against Women International
University of Massachusetts School
  of Nursing
Amherst, Massachusetts 01003

Oncology Nursing Society
501 Holiday Drive
Pittsburgh, Pennsylvania 15220

Respiratory Nursing Society
5700 Old Orchard Road
Skokie, Illinois 60077-1057

Society for Education and Research
  in Psychiatric-Mental Health
  Nursing
437 Twin Bay Drive
Pensacola, Florida 32534

Society of Gastroenterology Nurses
  and Associates, Inc.
1070 Sibley Tower
Rochester, New York 14604

Society of Otorhinolaryngology
  and Head/Neck Nurses
116 Canal Street, Suite A
New Smyrna Beach, Florida 32168

Society of Pediatric Nurses
7250 Parkway Drive, Suite 510
Hanover, Maryland 21076

Society of Rogerian Scholars
P.O. Box 1195, Canal Street Station
New York, New York 10013-0867

Society for Vascular Nursing
309 Winter Street
Norwood, Massachusetts 02062

Transcultural Nursing Society
College of Nursing & Health
Madonna University
36600 Schoolcraft Road
Livonia, Michigan 48150

**Visiting Nurse Associations
of America**
3801 E. Florida Avenue, Suite 900
Denver, Colorado 80210

....
....
....
....
....
....
APPENDIX C
....

State Boards of Nursing

Alabama
Alabama Board of Nursing
P.O. Box 303900
Montgomery, Alabama 36130-8900

Alaska
Alaska Board of Nursing
P.O. Box 110806
Juneau, Alaska 99811

American Samoa
American Samoa Health Service
Regulatory Board
LBJ Tropical Medical Center
Pago Pago, American Samoa 96799

Arizona
Arizona State Board of Nursing
1651 E. Morten Avenue, Suite 150
Phoenix, Arizona 85020

Arkansas
Arkansas State Board of Nursing
University Tower Building,
    Suite 800
1123 South University
Little Rock, Arkansas 72204

California
California Board of Registered Nursing
P.O. Box 944210
Sacramento, California 94244-2100

Colorado
Colorado Board of Nursing
1560 Broadway, Suite 670
Denver, Colorado 80202

Connecticut
Connecticut Board of Examiners
    for Nursing
150 Washington Street
Hartford, Connecticut 06106

Delaware
Delaware Board of Nursing
Margaret O'Neill Building
P.O. Box 1401
Dover, Delaware 19903

District of Columbia
District of Columbia Board of Nursing
614 H Street N.W.
Washington, D.C. 20001

Florida
Florida Board of Nursing
111 Coastline Drive East,
    Suite 516
Jacksonville, Florida 32202

Georgia
Georgia Board of Nursing
166 Pryor Street S.W.
Atlanta, Georgia 30303

Guam
Guam Board of Examiners
P.O. Box 2816
Agana, Guam 96910

Hawaii
Hawaii Board of Nursing
P.O. Box 3469
Honolulu, Hawaii 96801

Idaho
Idaho Board of Nursing
P.O. Box 83720
Boise, Idaho 83720-0061

Illinois
Illinois Department of Professional
    Regulation
320 West Washington Street
Springfield, Illinois 62786

**Illinois Department of Professional
    Regulation**
100 West Randolph, Suite 9-300
Chicago, Illinois 60601

Indiana
Indiana State Board of Nursing
Health Professions Bureau
402 West Washington Street,
Room #041
Indianapolis, Indiana 46204

Iowa
Iowa Board of Nursing
State Capitol Complex
1223 East Court Avenue
Des Moines, Iowa 50319

Kansas
Kansas State Board of Nursing
Landon State Office Building
900 S.W. Jackson, Suite 551-S
Topeka, Kansas 66612-1230

Kentucky
Kentucky Board of Nursing
312 Wittington Parkway,
    Suite 300
Louisville, Kentucky, 40222-5172

Louisiana
Louisiana State Board of Nursing
912 Pere Marquette Building
150 Baronne Street
New Orleans, Louisiana 70112

Maine
Maine State Board of Nursing
State House Station #158
Augusta, Maine 04333-0158

Maryland
Maryland Board of Nursing
4140 Patterson Avenue
Baltimore, Maryland 21215-2299

Massachusetts
Massachusetts Board of Registration
    in Nursing
Leverett Saltonstall Building
100 Cambridge Street, Room 1519
Boston, Massachusetts 02202

Michigan
Bureau of Occupational
    & Professional Regulation
Michigan Department of Commerce
Ottawa Towers North
611 West Ottawa
Lansing, Michigan 48933

Minnesota
Minnesota Board of Nursing
2700 University Avenue, West 108
St. Paul, Minnesota 55114

Mississippi
Mississippi Board of Nursing
239 N. Lamar Street, Suite 401
Jackson, Mississippi 39201

Missouri
Missouri State Board of Nursing
P.O. Box 656
Jefferson City, Missouri 65102

Montana
Montana State Board of Nursing
111 North Jackson
P.O. Box 200513
Helena, Montana 59620-0513

Nebraska
Bureau of Examining Boards
Nebraska Department of Health
P.O. Box 95007
Lincoln, Nebraska 68509

Nevada
Nevada State Board of Nursing
P.O. Box 46886
Las Vegas, Nevada 89114

New Hampshire
New Hampshire Board of Nursing
Health & Welfare Building
6 Hazen Drive
Concord, New Hampshire 03301-6527

New Jersey
New Jersey Board of Nursing
P.O. Box 45010
Newark, New Jersey 07101

New Mexico
New Mexico Board of Nursing
4206 Louisiana Blvd N.E., Suite A
Albuquerque, New Mexico 87109

New York
New York Board of Nursing
State Education Department
Cultural Education Center,
    Room 3023
Albany, New York 12230

North Carolina
North Carolina Board of Nursing
P.O. Box 2129
Raleigh, North Carolina 27602

North Dakota
North Dakota Board of Nursing
919 South 7th Street, Suite 504
Bismarck, North Dakota 58504-5881

Ohio
Ohio Board of Nursing
77 South High Street
Columbus, Ohio 43266-0316

Oklahoma
Oklahoma Board of Nursing
2915 North Classen Blvd, Suite 524
Oklahoma City, Oklahoma 73106

Oregon
Oregon State Board of Nursing
800 N.E. Oregon Street, Box 25
Suite 465
Portland, Oregon 97232

Pennsylvania
Pennsylvania State Board of Nursing
P.O. Box 2649
Harrisburg, Pennsylvania 17105-2649

Puerto Rico
Commonwealth of Puerto Rico
Board of Nurse Examiners
Call Box 10200
Santurce, Puerto Rico 00903

Rhode Island
Rhode Island Board of Nurse
    Registration & Nursing
    Education
Cannon Health Building
Three Capitol Hill, Room 101
Providence, Rhode Island 02908-5097

South Carolina
South Carolina State Board of Nursing
220 Executive Center Drive, Suite 220
Columbia, South Carolina 29210

South Dakota
South Dakota Board of Nursing
3307 South Lincoln Avenue
Sioux Falls, South Dakota 57105-5224

Tennessee
Tennessee State Board of Nursing
283 Plus Park Boulevard
Nashville, Tennessee 37217-1010

Texas
Texas Board of Nurse Examiners
P.O. Box 140466
Austin, Texas 78714

Utah
Utah State Board of Nursing
Division of Occupational &
    Professional Licensing
P.O. Box 45805
Salt Lake City, Utah 84145-0805

Vermont
Vermont State Board of Nursing
109 State Street
Montpelier, Vermont 05609-1106

Virgin Islands
Virgin Islands Board of Nurse
    Licensure
P.O. Box 4247, Veterans Drive Station
St. Thomas, U.S. Virgin Islands 00803

Virginia
Virginia Board of Nursing
6606 West Broad Street
Richmond, Virginia 23230

Washington
Washington State Nursing Care
    Quality Assurance Commission
Department of Health
P.O. Box 47864
Olympia, Washington 98504-7864

West Virginia
West Virginia Board of Examiners
    for Registered Professional
    Nurses
101 Dee Drive
Charleston, West Virginia 25311-1620

Wisconsin
Wisconsin Department of Regulation
    & Licensing
1400 East Washington Avenue
P.O. Box 8935
Madison, Wisconsin 53708-8935

Wyoming
Wyoming State Board of Nursing
Barrett Building
2301 Central Avenue
Cheyenne, Wyoming 82002

....
....
....
....
....
....
INDEX
....